THE AIDS COVER-UP?

GENE ANTONIO

THE AIDS COVER-UP?

The Real and Alarming
Facts about AIDS

IGNATIUS PRESS   SAN FRANCISCO

Second edition, with supplement

Cover by Marcia Ryan

© 1986, 1987 Gene Antonio
ISBN 0-89870-128-7 (HB)
ISBN 0-89870-129-5 (PB)
Library of Congress catalogue number 86-81935
Printed in the United States of America

When this book was first published in September, 1987, many reviewers called its assertions extreme, alarmist and unfounded. Yet almost every week since its original publication some team of researchers or medical scientists has confirmed the results of Gene Antonio's extensive investigations.

Although the amount of data on AIDS is increasing at an accelerated pace as public health officials and scientists themselves are recognizing the dimensions of this pandemic, the most recent findings only confirm Antonio's original conclusions. If anything, they show Antonio's evaluation of the extent and danger of this epidemic to have been too conservative.

In this second edition, therefore, it has not been necessary to revise the original material. But a supplement has been added to indicate the most recent major findings and to show how they confirm Antonio's original thesis.

— *The Publisher*

Dedicated to Atyam

CONTENTS

FOREWORD

Dr. William A. Haseltine, a leading AIDS researcher at the Harvard Medical School in Boston has warned that

> the AIDS epidemic will produce an "enormous" and "frightening" effect on world health that public health officials may be "relatively powerless to contain".
>
> Dr. Haseltine . . . painted one of the most frightening pictures of AIDS yet put forth by any prominent scientist. He noted that perhaps a million people in the United States, and conceivably 20 million worldwide, had already been infected with the virus, even though only a small percentage had yet become sick.
>
> "We must be prepared to anticipate that the vast majority of those now infected will ultimately, over a period of five to ten years, develop life-threatening illness", he said.
>
> The Harvard scientist also warned that "outstanding citizens" in New York City who visit prostitutes have a one in five chance of contracting the virus and taking it home to infect their wives.
>
> Even the blood supply is "not entirely safe", despite new screening tests, he said, and perhaps 2,000 cases of infection each year can be expected from contaminated blood donations. Noting that chlamydia, a venereal disease, had infected twenty percent to thirty percent of the college women tested in some studies, Dr. Haseltine said it seemed likely that the AIDS virus, also sexually transmitted, "may reach similar high levels". (P. M. Boffey, "Top Official and Expert Urge More AIDS Funds", *New York Times* [27 September 1985])

The AIDS Cover-Up? is a book destined to stir up no small amount of controversy. Whether or not one agrees with its conclusions, it must be affirmed that the author has accurately compiled a vast amount of research drawn from quality medical sources. It is extraordinarily informative and draws attention to important issues which need to be addressed.

One of the most noteworthy aspects of the work is that facts and statements of experts in the field have generally been presented dispassionately. It is written in a scholarly yet readable manner. Much of the material is left open-ended so as to act as a catalyst for further discussion and analysis.

The United States and other nations of the world are facing a health crisis of catastrophic proportions. One thing is certain: the AIDS epidemic is not simply going to go away. Considering the enormous magnitude of the AIDS epidemic, the information presented in this book needs to reach as broad an audience as possible. Both medical personnel and the general public will benefit from considering the facts it presents.

E. Robert Geiger, M.D., F.A.C.S.

INTRODUCTION

THE DANGERS ARE REAL

Infection with the AIDS virus is potentially lethal to all men, women and children irrespective of lifestyle or sexual activity.[1]
— Dr. John Seale, eminent British venereologist.

AIDS is no longer someone else's problem. Contrary to optimistic rumors, the AIDS epidemic is not leveling off. In 1986 more persons have been diagnosed with the disease than in all previous years (1978-1985) combined.[2] Those diagnosed as having AIDS represent only the tip of the iceberg. Between two and three million Americans are estimated to be permanently infected with the AIDS virus.

Dr. James Curran of the Centers for Disease Control notes:

> . . . in many areas, the number of persons infected with the AIDS virus is at least one hundred times greater than reported cases of AIDS.[3]

In his July 22, 1985, testimony before Congress, Dr. Dani Bolognesi of the Duke University Medical Center asserted that two million Americans were estimated to already have become permanently infected with the AIDS virus and to be at risk of developing the disease. The number of those infected, he averred, "is expected to double each year". Every day, thousands of persons are becoming newly infected.[4] The ranks of those contracting AIDS virus infection include men, women and children from a variety of backgrounds.

Unfortunately for society, there has been a consistent campaign of disinformation about the AIDS virus on the part of many public health officials and the media. Key facts regarding the nature of AIDS, its related conditions and its means of transmission have been glossed over and obscured.

Practical measures which could have helped stave off rapid spread of the virus throughout the population still have not been taken. This has left many people unnecessarily vulnerable to AIDS virus infection and uncertain about what steps to take in order to safeguard themselves and their loved ones.

As the death toll from AIDS virus infection mounts, there will be increasing demands for action to halt its massive spread. The public has a right to know all the pertinent information about this dangerous contagious disorder. Practical strategies for stopping this devastating epidemic must be based on objective data, not emotionalism.

This book examines the underlying ethical and legislative rationale which has fostered conditions encouraging AIDS virus spread and undermined attempts to halt its growth. It is designed to enable the discerning reader to determine which methods would be most effective in avoiding AIDS virus infection personally and preventing its continued widespread dissemination.

CHAPTER ONE

DESIGN FOR DISASTER—
HOW THE AIDS VIRUS OPERATES

*This system is very potent in permitting viruses to repro-
duce at a ferocious rate. It's one reason this is such a
devastating disease. It's one of the reasons this virus
can be transmitted so easily from person to person.* [1]
  — Dr. William Haseltine, AIDS researcher, the Dana-Farber
  Cancer Institute, Harvard University.

How AIDS Started among Humans

Present research suggests that AIDS made its initial
lethal intrusion into the human population in Africa.
The virus has been found in African green monkeys and
is similar to a class of viruses found in sheep.[2]

It has been speculated that humans initially became
infected through animal bites, eating tainted meat or
bestiality.[3] The virus then may have been passed on to
other humans via sexual contact and possibly by rituals
involving tattooing or scarring of the skin. Biting insects, such as mosquitoes, have also been cited as a
factor.[4]

The patterns of transmission of the AIDS virus are
highly similar to those of hepatitis B.[5] This has important implications for the spread of the AIDS virus. In
addition to routes involving sexual transmission and
multi-use of unsterilized needles, other modes of transmission may be involved. The eminent British venereologist Dr. John Seale notes:

1

... [both hepatitis B and the AIDS virus] are also easily transmitted by the close, non-sexual contact with infected cuts, sores, and abrasions, and the blood or serum of other people. ... [6]

The Introduction of AIDS Virus Infection to the United States

Although not recognized as such at the time, cases of AIDS virus infection in the United States first appeared during the middle and late 1970s.[7] The lengthy incubation period of the virus indicates that infection with the AIDS virus had actually begun occurring several years previously, possibly around 1970 or before. In the May 21, 1982, *Mortality and Morbidity Weekly Report,* the Centers for Disease Control reported:

> Since October of 1981, cases of persistent, generalized lymphadenopathy [swollen lymph glands]—not attributable [at that time] to previously identified causes—among homosexual males had been reported to the Centers for Disease Control (CDC) by physicians in several major metropolitan areas in the United States. These reports were prompted by an awareness generated by ongoing CDC and state investigations of other emerging health problems among homosexual males.[8]

Just how long the AIDS virus has been at work among humans is a very controversial issue. In her book *Gay Men's Health: A Guide to the AID Syndrome and Other Sexually Transmitted Diseases,* Dr. Jeanne Kassler cites a thought-provoking case which may indicate that the syndrome has been affecting humans far longer than realized:

Since the epidemic of immune suppression is new, scientists are wondering whether they may be dealing with a new virus. It is of interest that a case similar to AIDS in many ways was reported in a British medical journal more than 20 years ago. In the *Lancet* of October 29, 1960, doctors described a young man with oral and anal ulcers who died rapidly of overwhelming Pneumocystis and CMV [cytomegalovirus] infection. On the surface at least, this sounds much like AIDS.[9]

Between 1976 and 1981, CDC-defined AIDS in the United States was linked almost exclusively with the practice of homosexuality. From January 1976 through July 1981, 94 percent (95/101) of the men with AIDS for whom sexual preference was known were homosexual or bisexual. Only one female case of AIDS had been diagnosed during that time.[10]

The correlation between the practice of homosexuality and occurrence of this syndrome was so strong that initially it was called GRID, the Gay Related Immunodeficiency Disease. In deference to intense lobbying efforts by homosexual medical activists and as the disease was spread to other groups, the title GRID was replaced by the more generic acronym AIDS, Acquired Immunodeficiency Syndrome.[11]

By 1982, the AIDS virus had spread out of its previous epidemiologic closet of confinement. Intravenous (IV) drug abusers, infants, hemophiliacs and Haitians had been diagnosed with the full-blown syndrome.[12]

THE U.S.-HAITI AIDS CONNECTION

Early in the course of the epidemic, it was speculated that Haiti had been a source of the spread of AIDS to the United States. Now, it appears the reverse was actually the case. In the July 14, 1984, issue of *Lancet,* researchers from Belgium, Zaire and the United States reported:

> We are unaware of any facts implicating either central Africa or Haitian immigrants from central Africa as the origin of the disease, and such speculation must be viewed with scepticism unless substantive data appear.[13]

An analysis by a specialist at the University of Southern California went even further:

> The association with Haiti has caused confusion. AIDS in the United States *antedated* that in Haiti, and the disease was probably *introduced* into the Haitian population by vacationing American homosexuals for whom the island was a fashionable resort in the late 1970s.
>
> Interestingly, Haitian born patients with AIDS are the only group in the United States in whom AIDS has become proportionately less prevalent compared with others at risk[14] [emphasis added].

Houses of male prostitution had been previously established by Western homosexuals visiting the island. Also, common Haitian folk-medicine practices involving the repeated use of unsterilized needles would guarantee the spread of AIDS virus in that country, once introduced by American homosexual tourists.

AIDS SPREAD IN EUROPE

Homosexual males have also formed the vanguard of AIDS virus spread in Europe. At first, almost 90 percent of all AIDS cases in Europe were reported among male homosexuals. From this group it has spread to blood transfusion recipients and IV-drug abusers.[15]

Exactly how and where the AIDS virus entered into humankind is a question which may never fully be resolved. The stark reality of the growing pandemic this rapidly reproducing virus has spawned is not, however, a moot issue. AIDS and related AIDS virus conditions are a permanent, unyielding enemy of the human race which are relentlessly spreading on a national and international scale into all segments of the population.

What AIDS Is

As the name implies, the Acquired Immunodeficiency Syndrome is best known for producing an inability of the body's immune system to ward off infections. It is known that a person acquires the full-blown disease or its precursor conditions by becoming infected with the AIDS virus. Infants born to infected mothers have acquired the disorder both in the womb, during and after birth.[16] The possibility of postnatal transmission of AIDS apart from sexual abuse is one of the most troubling issues raised by researchers.

Dr. Gene M. Shearer, of the National Cancer Institute, has cautioned that:

> If an AIDS infectious agent exists and is opportunistic, with the syndrome becoming fully expressed only in immune-deficient persons, then infants with environmental exposure to the AIDS agent should be very susceptible.[17]

The AIDS Virus Multiplies Rapidly

The agent which causes AIDS is a retrovirus designated HTLV–III/LAV (human T-cell lymphotropic retrovirus/ lymphadenopathy-associated virus).[18] The AIDS virus reproduces with rapidity.

> "The kind of readout of genetic information we see in this system is absolutely astounding", asserts Dr. William Haseltine, a prominent investigator at Harvard's Dana-Farber Cancer Institute. "Nobody would have thought this level of transcription [gene activity] was possible before we did these studies. We were shocked. It's about 1,000 times faster than the . . . genes we know about.
>
> "This system is very potent in permitting viruses to replicate at a ferocious rate. It's one reason this is such a devastating disease. It's one of the reasons this virus can be transmitted so easily from person to person."[19]

According to Dr. Luc Montagnier, the eminent French AIDS researcher who, concurrently with Dr. Robert Gallo, discovered the HTLV–III/LAV retrovirus as the AIDS agent, this has dire import in terms of the possibility of vaccine development and potential new routes of AIDS spread:

> *The potential for genetic variation is perhaps the greatest danger in the future of the AIDS epidemic.* It will make it difficult to design efficient vaccines protective against all strains, and a further change of the virus in its tropism [ability to infect types of cells] and *ways of transmission cannot be excluded*[20] [emphasis added].

Researchers from the World Health Organization Collaborating Centre on AIDS have reported:

The possibility of a *mutant strain* [of AIDS], with particular pathogenic properties, causing *a new epidemic phenomenon* is consistent with the observations of Zairian investigators who have reported an outbreak of cryptoccocal meningitis in Kinshasa [Zaire].[21]

The extraordinary reproductive capacity of the AIDS virus makes bodily invasion with even a minute amount of the virus a matter of grave concern. According to Dr. John Seale,

... it is probable that, as with so many viraemic diseases, *a single virion* [virus] *introduced directly into the blood will regularly transmit infection*[22] [emphasis added].

This means that healthy medical workers with AIDS-tainted needle-stick injuries may be susceptible to AIDS infection. The incubation period in previously healthy persons appears to be longer than in persons in high-risk groups who have been infected with larger doses of the virus and frequently are beset with immune dysfunction prior to infection.[23] Thus needle-stick injuries in non-high-risk-group persons may take much longer to result in overt AIDS infection.

After infection occurs, the AIDS virus travels throughout various parts of the body. The AIDS virus has been isolated from plasma, serum, saliva, tears, semen, urine, cerebrospinal fluid and brain tissue.[24] In addition, it has recently been found in vaginal secretions.[25]

It may, in fact be found in a variety of tissues, as described by Dr. Jeffrey Laurence, an AIDS researcher at New York Hospital-Cornell Medical Center:

Other cells outside the blood may also serve as reservoirs [for the AIDS virus]: the endothelial cells lining the blood and lymphatic vessels, the cells of epithelium (skin and related tissues), the glial cells of the nervous system and nerve cells themselves.[26]

It should be noted that if, as it appears, the AIDS virus invades epithelial cells, this indicates the potential for spread through so-called casual means of transmission. Other viruses, such as hepatitis A and influenza viruses, are spread through inclusion in epithelial cells. Dr. Laurence also contends that the virus is likely secreted in sweat.[27]

How the AIDS Virus Operates

The AIDS virus has two known major means of causing death: indirect and direct.

INDIRECT MEANS OF AIDS DEATH

The most highly publicized aspect of the AIDS virus is its penchant for attacking and disabling the white blood cells which normally ward off infection. These white blood cells, called helper T-cells, normally serve to activate other cells which produce antibodies that attack invading organisms.

When the AIDS virus invades these white blood cells, their ability to defend against infection is seriously impaired. The helper T-cells lose their normal role and become AIDS virus factories. In the process, the T-cells are gradually destroyed, and as they disappear the main initiator of the immune response is lost. This effectively devastates the immune system.

In a recent *New York Magazine* article presumptuously entitled "The Last Word on Avoiding AIDS", the author declares flatly: "People don't die of AIDS. They die of other diseases they can't fight off."[28] However, contrary to similar statements, widely propounded in much of the media and press, researchers have known for over a year that

> the AIDS virus can kill by causing brain disease without any opportunistic infection and without immune suppression.[29]

The AIDS virus per se destroys cells in the brain and causes progressive brain disease (AIDS virus encephalopathy).[30] In the July 1985 issue of *Cell,* researchers from Harvard's Dana-Farber Cancer Institute reported: "The HTLV–III LTR [Long Terminal Repeat] directs gene expression in human lymphoid and nonlymphoid cells. . . . "[31] Dr. Robert Gallo, the American researcher who co-discovered the AIDS virus, states that the AIDS virus

> . . . is neurotropic as well as lymphotropic . . . studies confirm that some cells of the brain contain HTLV–III and suggest that these cells are not of lymphocyte origin.[32]

These findings indicate that the AIDS virus resides and reproduces in cells in the nervous system as well as in the lymphocytes in the immune system. Cases of AIDS virus-induced progressive brain disease appeared in New York over a year ago.[33] Medical reports indicate that AIDS-induced brain disease is one of the most significant aspects of AIDS infection. Researchers from Memorial Sloan-Kettering Cancer Center in New York have found that "The retrovirus responsible for AIDS commonly infects the central nervous system. . . ."[34]

The Three Stages of AIDS Infection

After entering the body, the time it takes for the AIDS virus to produce deadly effects varies among individuals. At present, there are three basic known stages which characterize persons infected with the virus.

STAGE ONE: ASYMPTOMATIC CARRIER STATE

The first stage is an asymptomatic carrier stage. The individual is infected with the virus but shows no detectable signs or symptoms. The person may appear in good health and may seemingly remain so for a number of years. The lack of outward manifestation of AIDS virus infection is deceptive.

The AIDS virus infiltrates the eyes, brain, lungs, liver, spleen, kidneys and other organs of infected persons, *including those who appear symptomless.*[35] It appears that the AIDS virus may be toxic to cells outside the brain and the immune system. The AIDS virus has been implicated in the degeneration of follicular dendritic cells in the spleen as well as those of the lymph nodes of mice after immunization.[36]

Persons carrying the AIDS virus, including those who have not yet developed visible symptoms, are able to infect others.

The demonstration of HTLV–III in the blood and semen of a healthy individual establishes an asymptomatic, virus-positive carrier state which may be important in the dissemination of HTLV–III, and consequently, AIDS.[37]

After infection occurs, the body begins "shedding" the AIDS virus, excreting it through various bodily secretions. This is why infected persons who have not yet developed symptoms are able to transmit the AIDS virus to others. In the furor over whether AIDS "victims"—i.e., actual diagnosed AIDS patients—should be quarantined, allowed to attend school, remain food handlers etc., a fundamental point has been largely ignored: *individuals who are infected with the AIDS virus but who demonstrate no visible symptoms are just as capable of spreading AIDS as patients with the full-blown syndrome.* [38]

Every individual who has fallen prey to infection with the AIDS virus is infected for the rest of his or her life. Dr. Gallo states: "Once infection by a retrovirus [i.e., AIDS] occurs, it is likely to be for the lifetime of the person." [39] There is no way of becoming "disinfected" from the virus. Once infected, a person remains permanently capable of passing the deadly agent on to others. Dr. Haseltine reiterates with finality:

> Once infected, a person remains infected for the rest of his life. Once infected a person is infectious. It is not safe to assume otherwise. [40]

In graphic personal terms, this means that, once a person becomes infected with the AIDS virus, he or she can never engage in intimate sexual activity without endangering the life of another person. According to regulations drafted by the CDC:

> Each person ... would have to be told ... that they cannot engage in sexual intercourse, kiss someone, or seek medical or dental care without exposing their partner or health care provider to this possibly deadly virus. [41]

The efficacy of condoms in preventing AIDS transmission is unproven.[42] "French" kissing, involving the exchange of infected saliva, should also be avoided. Dr. Slaff states: "Symptomless carriers . . . are putting every sexual contact at risk."[43]

Conception by an infected parent can mean a terrible death sentence for the developing infant.

> Among children there is a substantial risk for transmission from parent to offspring, particularly in the prenatal and perinatal period.[44]

Soon a total of 35,000 AIDS cases will have been reported by the CDC. This figure grossly underrates the immense scope of the problem. Margaret Heckler, former Secretary of Health and Human Services, stated at the International Conference on AIDS in April of 1985:

> Acquired immunodeficiency syndrome (AIDS) kills. The danger of the syndrome's deadly thrust is compounded because, like the iceberg's mammoth underwater size, the long gestation period of AIDS gives no initial warning of the omnipresent danger.[45]

In a paper presented at the same Conference, Dr. James Curran of the CDC reported:

> It is reasonable to assume that in many areas the number of persons infected with HTLV–III/LAV is *at least one hundred times higher* than that of reported cases of AIDS. Because HTLV–III/LAV is a retrovirus, persistent, even *lifelong* infection would be expected[46] [emphasis added].

This means that in the near future there could be at least 3,500,000 persons permanently infected with the AIDS virus in the United States. All of these individuals are capable of transmitting the virus to others.

The second stage of AIDS virus infection occurs when an infected individual begins to manifest symptoms which can include sudden unexplained weight loss, drenching night sweats, persistent diarrhea, swelling of the lymph nodes in the armpits and groin, chronic fatigue and/or psychogenic disturbances. This has been called the AIDS related complex (ARC) or the pre-AIDS syndrome.

Dubbing this second stage of AIDS virus infection the 'pre-'AIDS syndrome is something of a misnomer. Persons developing ARC are critically infected with the AIDS virus. They are beset with a wide range of grave health problems. Dr. James Slaff, Medical Investigator at the National Institutes of Health, states that there are over 50 clinical manifestations of ARC.[47]

As the AIDS virus begins to invade cells in the brain and central nervous system, signs of nascent dementia develop. These include chronic memory loss, loss of muscular control, seizures, mutism (inability to speak coherently or at all) and severe psychiatric disturbances.[48]

An example of the severe neurological/psychiatric complications which occur during this stage was reported in the August 17, 1985 issue of *Lancet:*

> ... CNS [central nervous system] and neuropsychiatric complications can occur in AIDS. Opportunistic infections ... are often responsible. A recent report suggests that *HTLV-III itself can infect neuronal matter to produce an encephalopathy* [brain disease], which may cause malaise, lethargy depression, personality change, confusion, headaches, seizures, ataxia [loss of muscular coordination], impaired short-term memory, and finally a dementia [organic brain degeneration]. ...
>
> We describe here a 22-year-old homosexual man who

presented with lymphadenopathy (swollen lymph glands—symptomatic of ARC) and psychiatric disturbance and was later discovered to be HTLV-III positive.

Three months after the lymphadenopathy was recognized he had a paranoid psychosis. He believed that he was in great danger of coming to harm and that he had superhuman powers given to him by God. His behavior was bizarre, at times childlike and attention seeking, at other times withdrawn. . . .

A year later he became ill again and tried to throw himself in front of two passing vehicles. He was mute and negativistic and was admitted to hospital. . . . After five days his behavior became more bizarre—he picked up objects with his mouth, refused to communicate, and had occasional outbursts of aggression. After treatment [with medication] he said he felt guilty and depressed. . . . He also admitted to third-person auditory hallucinations several days earlier. He was fully oriented but had some difficulty concentrating. His memory for past events was good and he correctly named four out of six items of a name and address at five minutes. . . .

In our patient no opportunistic infection or Kaposi's sarcoma was identified, which excludes a diagnosis of AIDS according to the Centers for Disease Control (CDC) criteria [49] [emphasis added].

The gravity of this second stage of AIDS infection should not be minimized. AIDS-induced brain disease is irreversible.[50]

Patients like the one above are suffering from severe complications related to AIDS infection. They are not included in the total number of AIDS cases reported by the CDC. At present, only persons diagnosed with "full-blown" AIDS are reported by the CDC. The number of persons with pre-AIDS or AIDS related complex (ARC), however, is estimated by some researchers to be ten times the number of full-blown AIDS cases.[51]

By the end of 1986, there will be approximately 350,000 persons suffering severe debilitating physical and mental illnesses as a result of AIDS infection who are not included in the total of AIDS cases reported by the CDC. Persons in this intermediate stage of AIDS infections are also capable of transmitting the AIDS virus to others.

STAGE THREE: FULL-BLOWN AIDS

In light of the progressive nature of AIDS-induced brain disease, the distinction between persons suffering with AIDS related complex (ARC) and what is officially defined as AIDS has become blurred. As noted above, AIDS-induced dementia without severe immune suppression or AIDS related disease is still not included in the category of full-blown AIDS.

The other diseases which beset persons in this stage are called opportunistic infections. They attack when the breakdown of the immune system leaves the body vulnerable. Infection by these disease agents frequently has occurred prior to the onset of AIDS virus infection. Normally the immune system would protect against their damaging effects, but as its capacity to defend against infection is impaired, these normally uncommon infections are given free rein to spread throughout the body.

The most frequently occurring opportunistic diseases during this terminal stage of AIDS include:

Pneumocystis carinii Pneumonia (PCP): a parasitic infection which infiltrates the lungs. Patients with PCP experience shortness of breath, sharp chest pains when inhaling deeply and a persistent, wheezing cough that is either dry or accompanied by small amounts of white sputum. A sense of suffocation develops as the infection permeates the lungs.

Kaposi's sarcoma (KS): a particularly invasive form of skin cancer which involves the internal organs. Unlike cancers which originate from a single malignant cell and then spread to other parts of the body, independent cancerous growths of KS occur in different areas even without metastasis. KS can develop in the lungs, lymph nodes, liver, stomach, spleen and intestines.

KS skin lesions, initially appearing as small purplish spots, can occur on the neck, armpits, eyes, mouth, torso, arms, legs and around the genital/anal area.[52]

Pneumocystis carinii Pneumonia and Kaposi's sarcoma are the most commonly occurring devastating diseases associated with AIDS, and these can occur concurrently and with other infections as well.[53]

Candidiasis: a fungal infection which produces a condition in the mouth known as thrush. Thrush is characterized by white patches like milk curds lining the mouth and tongue. Along with swollen lymph glands, candidiasis is one of the most common early warning signs of AIDS. This infection can spread to the esophagus and into the bloodstream and central nervous system. Patients develop chest pain and difficulty in swallowing.

Cytomegalovirus (CMV): a devastating viral infection which commonly attacks the lungs and can spread throughout the body. CMV necrotizing retinitis can cause blindness. Much of the adult population in this country have been infected with CMV infection at one time or another. As with other opportunistic infections, the consequences in immunologically-impaired AIDS patients are much more serious than usual. Among homosexuals, persistent repeated reinfection with CMV, often including different strains, has been implicated in the high rate of Kaposi's sarcoma occuring mainly in their group.

Herpes simplex (HSV): causes painful, severe ulcers around the mouth and perianal areas. Colitis may also occur with bleeding, cramps and weight loss. In AIDS patients, HSV infections may disseminate with serious and often fatal consequences.

Herpes zoster: causes skin eruptions commonly known as "shingles". In AIDS patients it may lead to oozing blisters and large black scabs over the infected areas, such as the mouth, nose and rectum.[54]

Toxoplasmosis: caused by *Toxoplasma gondii*, a small intracellular parasite which is often found in cat feces. Though normally a mild asymptomatic infection in persons with intact immune systems, it can be a fulminating and disseminated infection in AIDS patients. It is most frequently found in AIDS patients in association with CNS symptoms such as headaches, severe lethargy, seizures, vomiting, fever and psychological disturbances. *T. gondii* CNS disturbances differ from encephalopathy induced by the direct attack of the AIDS virus on brain tissue.)

Cryptosporidiosis: an intestinal disease caused by a protozoan often found in farm livestock, dogs, cats and other animals. It is spread by direct contact with infected feces. In patients with AIDS, it may cause a devastating, cholera-like syndrome, producing as much as ten liters per day of diarrhea. This leads to severe dehydration and malnutrition, causing drastic weight loss.

Unlike some of the other opportunistic infections whose symptoms may be alleviated, at least temporarily, by treatment, cryptosporidiosis in AIDS patients has proven "refractory to all therapeutic modalities".[55]

Cryptococcosis — a fungal infection which, in AIDS patients, may cause diffuse meningitis. Symptoms include stupor, mental disturbances and personality changes, accompanied by severe headaches, double vision and facial weakness.[56] (Note that this also differs from direct AIDS virus-induced encephalopathy resulting in dementia.)

Newly Recognized Complications of AIDS Virus Infection

Oral "Hairy" Leukoplakia:

An outbreak of a new form of oral leukoplakia, found principally on the borders of the tongue, is reported in male homosexuals in the San Francisco area.... Hairy leukoplakia appears to be a new entity found, as yet exclusively, in the mouths of male homosexuals....

Hairy leukoplakia appears to be associated with the papilloma virus [found in venereal warts, common among homosexuals] and a virus of the herpes group....

There is evidence that the patients are immuno-suppressed and that a substantial proportion progress to AIDS.[57]

Oral viral hairy leukoplakia of the tongue appears as raised white areas of thickening on the tongue, usually on the lateral border. The lesions may not respond to traditional anti-fungal therapy and appear to have unusual virologic features. Candida has been reported on the surface of the HL lesions. A number of viruses, including papilloma, herpes and Epstein-Barr virus [EBV], have been identified ... from the lesions. *HL was first identified in San Francisco in 1981*[58] [emphasis added].

Malignant lymphoma: this virulent form of lymphoma associated with AIDS virus infections has been found to attack extranodal sites in the central nervous system, rectum and/or anus in persons at risk for AIDS.

> HTLV-III associated lymphomas occurring in members of those groups at risk for AIDS are unusual in a clinical sense, even compared with similar high-grade lymphoma cases occurring in HTLV-III negative heterosexuals. . . . Lymphoma primary to the anus and/or rectum is highly unusual . . . [as is] the high incidence of central nervous system involvement.
>
> Recent information from the large population areas of San Francisco, Los Angeles, Houston, and New York indicate that these lymphomas are not sporadic, but may, in fact, represent another facet of the current epidemic of acquired immunodeficiency syndrome (AIDS).[59]

The occurrence of B–Cell Lymphoma in two monogamously paired homosexual males, only one of whom had severe immune suppression, has also been reported.[60] The respected British medical journal *Lancet* reports:

> There is growing evidence that male homosexuals are at increased risk of acquiring aggressive malignant lymphomas. . . . About 50% of patients have pre-existing AIDS or AIDS-related conditions. . . . The prognosis is dismal: response to chemotherapy is poor, relapse rates are high, and mean survival is less than one year.[61]

Tuberculosis: Although the rate of TB had been declining in the United States since the 1950s, the disease is making a dramatic comeback due to AIDS, according to federal and local officials.

> The officials note that areas with the largest increase in tuberculosis, including New York City and California, are identical to those with the highest rates of AIDS. They say new research indicates that the onset of tuber-

culosis may provide an early warning of AIDS in high risk groups. . . . "It is of great concern both for this country and for the rest of the world", says Dr. Dixie Snider Jr., director of the division of tuberculosis control for the federal Centers for Disease Control. . . .

Tuberculosis, however, is not considered an "opportunistic infection" because it is much more virulent than other infections associated with AIDS and has the potential to strike beyond AIDS victims, Snider said.

Snider said that AIDS victims often contract a form of tuberculosis that affects organs other than the lungs, such as the kidneys, bones, lymph nodes and brain. Thus, he said, it is important that TB be diagnosed accurately "because it is contagious and can be transmitted".[62]

Simultaneous tuberculous brain abscess and toxoplasmosis of the brain have been reported in the course of AIDS infection.[63] This also differs from direct destruction of brain tissue by the AIDS virus.

Full-Blown AIDS Leaves No Survivors

The survival prospects for those who move on to stage three of AIDS virus infection are extremely poor. More than half of those initially diagnosed with full-blown AIDS will be dead within eighteen months; more than 70 percent will be dead within two years.[64] Virtually no one who has developed the syndrome was alive five years later.

Reports of the ratio of AIDS patients who have died to those still alive can give the erroneous impression that a significant percentage of those diagnosed may survive the disease. For example:

The first 10,000 cases of acquired immune deficiency syndrome had been reported to the Centers for Disease

Control by last May 4. By Monday, January 6, 1986, the
total had risen to 16,138, with 8,220 deaths.[65]

In reality, the number of those living reflects cases
which have been recently identified. Over the long
term, the evidence is all too clear: full-blown AIDS is
terminal.

WHAT PERCENTAGE OF THOSE INFECTED WITH THE AIDS VIRUS WILL DIE FROM AIDS?

For some time it had been conservatively speculated
that from 10 to 20 percent of the persons initially
infected with the AIDS virus (Stage 1) would go on to
develop severe immune deficiency and fall prey to the
infections accompanying it (Stage 3). The fate of the
other 80 to 90 percent of those infected is a looming
question which has been left relatively unaddressed.
The lengthy incubation period of the virus made it
difficult to determine their ultimate prognosis. Mounting scientific evidence indicates that the long-term outlook for all persons infected with the AIDS virus is
much worse than was anticipated.

The notion that the AIDS virus operates solely by
initiating the destruction of the immune system is grossly
inaccurate and misleading. It is incontrovertibly established that the AIDS virus can kill directly rather than
solely by the effects of immune suppression.

AIDS-INDUCED BRAIN DISEASE—THE ULTIMATE KILLER

Media attention has been scant regarding the ability of
the AIDS virus to destroy brain cells apart from diseases related to immune deficiency. Nevertheless, CNS
tropism of the AIDS virus (its ability to infect cells in

the central nervous system) is one of the most crucial factors in determining the long-range course of AIDS infection.

Scientists have discovered that the AIDS virus travels into the cerobrospinal fluid and the tissues of the brain. Once there, it reproduces, killing the infected cells. The resulting progressive brain tissue destruction affects the thought processes (leading to dementia) and coordination of vital bodily functions. This differs from opportunistic infection of the brain which results from immune suppression.

The ability of the AIDS virus to cause brain destruction has helped uncover its true nature. Scientists now have a disease model more similar to AIDS (but without the immune suppression) which may help our understanding of the long-term course of AIDS virus infection.

A type of virus infection found in sheep, the maedi-visna virus, has some striking parallels to AIDS infection in humans. Infection with the maedi-visna virus causes a lung disease in sheep similar to the rare type of pneumonia found in AIDS patients. Infection by the visna virus also kills sheep by causing progressive brain disease without producing immune deficiency.

The AIDS virus and the visna virus belong to the family of lentiviruses. These lentiviruses (the name is derived from the Latin *lentus* — "slow") are called slow viruses because they frequently have a lengthy incubation period before symptoms develop. Apart from the new human form, only three other species of lentiviruses are known: the lentiviruses causing maedi-visna in sheep, infectious anemia in horses and encephalitis-arthritis in goats.

After the AIDS retrovirus was isolated, it was incorrectly assumed to be an oncornavirus [associated with cancer] for nearly two years. The suggestion that the early patients with AIDS represented the start of a pandemic of a slow virus disease in man was ignored for almost two years.[66]

Finally, in January of 1985, a report in *Science* clearly demonstrated that HTLV-III had been found in the brains of children and adults with AIDS encephalopathy. The report stated that HTLV-III appeared to be related to the visna lentivirus causing chronic degenerative brain disease in sheep.[67]

At the International Conference on AIDS in Atlanta in April of 1985, Dr. Robert Gallo, the American researcher who along with Dr. Luc Montagnier discovered the AIDS virus, reported:

Parallels of HTLV-III and lentiviruses . . . suggest they likely belong in the same virus category.[68]

Dr. Montagnier, of the Pasteur Institute in France, concurred that the AIDS virus should be classified as a lentivirus.

The retrovirus associated with lymphadenopathy [ARC] and AIDS is *the prototype of a new group of human retroviruses,* different from the HTLV group. Its genome structure suggests that *it represents the human equivalent of lentiviruses.*[69] [emphasis added].

Though not receiving wide publicity by public health officials or the media, the fact that HTLV-III is a lentivirus is of utmost importance in determining the long-range effects of AIDS infection and modes of AIDS virus transmission.

THE GRAVE PROGNOSIS OF AIDS INFECTION:
ALL PERSONS INFECTED MAY DIE

1. *Lentiviruses are lethal.*

After the AIDS virus was isolated, it was mistakenly thought to be part of the family of oncornaviruses which cause leukemia in humans. These oncornaviruses had been widely researched because of their association with cancer. As a result, there was a guarded optimism in some quarters about the possibility of finding a cure or vaccine for AIDS. It was, however, well-known in medical circles that no vaccine had ever before been developed against an RNA virus.

The realization that HTLV-III is a lentivirus further dimmed hopes of the possibility of developing a cure or vaccine. These lentiviruses are extremely virulent and complex. Little is understood about their role in disease. Infections with these slow-acting viruses in animals have proved completely resistant to any type of treatment or vaccine. Writing in the *Journal of the Royal Society of Medicine,* Dr. Seale comments:

> The lentiviruses have been largely neglected because they appeared irrelevant to disease in man and could not be transmitted to small laboratory animals. In domestic animals lentivirus infections have proved so lethal and unresponsive to treatment, and vaccines have proved so useless, that slaughter of infected animals has been the universal means of control.[70]

The realization that the AIDS virus is part of the deadly and little understood family of lentiviruses dashed the hopes that a vaccine or cure might soon be forthcoming. Dr. Haseltine of Harvard, states that in attempting to comprehend AIDS:

we have moved from being explorers in a canoe to explorers with a small sail on the vast sea of what we do not know.[71]

The overwhelming mortality rate of lentivirus infection has cast a dark shadow on the future of all those infected with AIDS. Dr. William Blattner and other researchers at the National Cancer Institute in Maryland assert:

We are at an early stage of the AIDS epidemic, and it is not unrealistic (judging from other human and animal retroviral models) to expect that long-term sequelae such as malignancy and chronic degenerative diseases may eventually occur in persons infected with HTLV-III virus.[72]

Along with a team of colleagues, Dr. Jay Levy of the Cancer Research Institute, University of California School of Medicine, San Francisco concluded:

The initial description in 1954 of these slow virus or lentivirus infections by Sigurdsson defined the acquired immunodeficiency syndrome: a long but predictable incubation period of months to years; an infectious agent that produces inapparent but progressive pathologic damage; and a protracted course, *generally ending in serious disease or death.*[73] [emphasis added].

2. *The AIDS lentivirus attacks the brain.*
The fact that HTLV-III is a slow acting virus which persistently infects cells throughout the brain has dire consequences. Among sheep, brain infection with the visna lentivirus results in the death of 100 percent of the animals after an asymptomatic period of one to six years, without producing any immune deficiency.[74]
Among humans, the AIDS virus also becomes imbedded in brain tissue and the cells of the central

nervous system. The virus then reproduces, irreversibly destroying the cells it infects. Dr. Slaff of the National Institutes of Health reports the case of a medical school teacher who developed dementia without any manifestation of ARC or full-blown AIDS. Viral replication of HTLV–III within the brain and cerebrospinal fluid was cited as the cause of death. Infants have been born without brains or with half brains. On autopsy, the AIDS virus was found in neurological tissue. A strange form of pancreatic cancer has also occurred in young individuals infected with the virus.[75] Cases like these have gone virtually unreported by the media.

The percentage of those infected with the AIDS virus who will succumb to disorders related to immune deficiency is large. The development of AIDS-induced brain disease will raise the overall mortality rate disastrously higher.

3. *The AIDS lentivirus has crossed the species barrier from animals to man.*

AIDS is a disease which has crossed over from one species, most probably the African green monkey, to another, namely mankind. Other diseases which have done this frequently do not harm the host animal but devastate the members of the new host species. Dr. Seale continues his analysis:

A highly significant consideration is that the AIDS virus is spreading as a virgin-soil epidemic throughout mankind after crossing the species barrier, probably from a green monkey.

A virus which successfully crosses the host-species barrier is often highly lethal to the new species, though harmless to its natural host. Infection with the myxomatosis virus causes harmless warts in the South American jungle rabbit, but the mortality exceeds 99% in the

European rabbit. The virus of African swine fever does not inconvenience the African wart-hog but it kills nearly all infected European pigs.[76]

An example of this deadly trans-species phenomenon has been evinced in Haiti. A recent outbreak of African swine fever killed hundreds of thousands of hogs and threatened the swine of other countries. This necessitated the slaughter of virtually every domestic pig on the Island.

Each of the above factors indicates that infection with the AIDS virus has lethal consequences. Combined, they indicate that there are dire long-range ramifications for all persons infected. Dr. James Slaff, Medical Investigator at the National Institutes of Health, estimates that between 30 and 45 percent of those infected will develop intermediate or full-blown AIDS within five years of becoming infected. The long-range prognosis beyond that, he predicts, is probably worse, "possibly much worse".[77] *Ultimately, infection with the AIDS virus may leave no survivors.*

This means that the majority—perhaps all—of the over two million persons already infected will probably die of AIDS-related disease. With the number of those presently infected expected to double this year to over four million,[78] the outlook for society becomes increasingly grim.

How Long Does It Take to Develop Symptoms after the AIDS Virus Invades the Body?

For those who go on to develop immune deficiency, the average time from initial infection to development of symptoms can vary from several weeks to five years or more.[79]

The lag time between initial infection and development of AIDS-induced brain disease may be ominously lengthy. By comparing the progress of other slow-acting infections of the brain, scientists estimate that the incubation period of AIDS-induced brain disease could range from two to thirty years, with a mean of fifteen years.

What Is the Life Expectancy of Persons Infected with the AIDS Virus?

A report from the Center for Infectious Diseases admits:

> The incubation period for AIDS is long. However, it may even be longer than our current estimates, because this infection has been only recently introduced into the United States and we may not have observed infected persons long enough for the longest-incubating cases to have developed. As a result, *our estimates of average incubation period may be short and our estimates of outcome may be low*[80] [emphasis added].

Dr. Seale notes:

> The eventual mortality following infection with a lentivirus like AIDS cannot be ascertained by direct observation till those recently infected have been followed well into the 21st century. In the case of maedi-visna lentivirus infection of sheep, the death rate reaches 100% within about two-thirds of the natural life span of the animal.[81]

The long-range outlook for AIDS lentivirus infection among humans is not good. Dr. Slaff comments:

> Although the model that best depicts the natural course of AIDS virus infection is uncertain, it appears that infected individuals face very serious long-term medical consequences. . . .

The five-year morbidity of AIDS virus infection is bad; *apparently all infected individuals will suffer significant medical consequences.* Even more distressing, the outlook for 10 years, 20 years, 30 years, and beyond is likely to be worse, possibly much worse[82] [emphasis added].

Why AIDS Is More Dangerous than Plague

Newly recognized animal viruses which have crossed to man in recent years and are blood borne have caused only limited epidemics. . . . They kill infected humans so quickly, and the immune response of those who survive kills the virus so rapidly after a transient infection, that they are incapable of sustaining an epidemic in man.

However, a new virus which produces a persistent viraemia for life, and causes a slow virus progressive brain disease after a mean incubation period of many years, would produce a self-sustaining epidemic. Indeed, it would produce a lethal pandemic throughout the crowded cities and villages of the Third World of a magnitude unparalleled in human history. This is what the AIDS virus is now doing.[83]

The astronomical growth of AIDS infection in the United States portends a destruction of human life exceeding casualties that would be suffered in a major war. AIDS is more dangerous and has far greater capacity for rapid spread than any other of the previous epidemics which have devastated large sections of humanity. With bubonic plague, cholera, smallpox and other epidemics, infected individuals manifest readily apparent symptoms (boils, dysentery, pox etc.) and can be readily identified and isolated before infecting others.

With AIDS, the lengthy asymptomatic carrier state which initially exists in the majority of those infected enables the disease to spread swiftly, unrealized, throughout vast numbers of the population. This is what the AIDS virus is now doing in the United States and other Western nations.

The present high level of AIDS infection in the United States, combined with the social and sexual mores of much of the population, indicates that developing nations are not alone in facing a pandemic of catastrophic proportions.

Summary Points and Implications

1. AIDS kills by two known means:
    a. Indirectly—by breaking down the immune system. This allows the development of various cancers and the occurrence of deadly infections from normally nonlethal organisms.
    b. Directly—by attacking and destroying brain cells. This results in progressive dementia.
2. Infection by the AIDS virus is a permanent condition. Entrance of only one virus into the body can result in infection. Once infected, a person remains so for the rest of his or her life.
3. Those infected asymptomatically are as capable of transmitting AIDS infection as those in the intermediate and end stages of the disease.
4. The contagious agent for AIDS is a slow-acting lentivirus. This indicates:
    a. AIDS infection will likely prove deadly to all persons infected through inducing progressive

     degenerative brain disease in those who do not
     first succumb to opportunistic infection.

  b. The adverse effects of AIDS infection can take
     many years to become manifest. This enables
     the epidemic to spread very rapidly.

5. The AIDS virus mutates very rapidly. New variant
   strains of the virus make vaccine development prospects bleak and could result in change in modes of
   transmission.

CHAPTER TWO:

HOW THE EPIDEMIC HAS SPREAD

Don't call us AIDS victims. AIDS is not my weakness. AIDS is my strength. [1]
— Paul Diamond, a homosexual activist diagnosed with Kaposi's sarcoma, *The Advocate*, May 28, 1985.

Why Homosexuals Have Been the Primary Group Affected Thus Far

In the United States, male homosexuals have comprised over three-fourths of all AIDS cases. The percentage of homosexuals among the total of all AIDS patients has remained relatively constant. In Europe, male homosexuals comprise over 85 percent of all AIDS cases.[2] The enormous prevalence of AIDS, along with several other grave communicable diseases endemic in this group, is not mere inexplicable chance. There are a number of major biological and social factors which have been distinctly linked with their spread.*

*The material in this section gives only a basic overview of the relationship between homosexual behavior and bodily trauma and diseases. For those in the medical, nursing, dental and legal professions, as well as other concerned parties requiring more extensive treatment of the subject, the following books are recommended: *Sexually Transmitted Diseases in Homosexual Men,* edited by David G. Ostrow, Terri A. Sandholzer and Yehudi M. Felman (Plenum Books, 1983) and *The Acquired Immune Deficiency Syndrome and Infections of Homosexual Men,* by Pearl Ma and Donald Armstrong (Yorke Medical Books, 1984).

Biological Factors in AIDS Spread
Among Homosexuals: The Hazards of Sodomy

DANGERS TO THE PASSIVE RECIPIENT

Among male homosexuals, sodomy or anal intercourse is the act substituted for heterosexual penile-vaginal coitus. This damaging practice provides ready access for the transmission of AIDS and other virulent infections.[3]

Physiologically, the rectum is designed for the expulsion of feces. When sodomy is performed, the peculiar forced inward expansion of the anal canal results in a tearing of the lining as well as bleeding anal fissures.[4]

Violent spasms of the bowel wall may occur as a reaction to the bodily intrusion. Colitis, a severe inflammation of the mucous membrane of the colon, often develops as sodomy is repeatedly engaged in. This disorder causes fever, malaise, painful wrenching cramps in the lower abdomen and eruptive diarrhea that commonly contains blood or leukocytes.[5] Along with anal fissure and syphilitic chancre, mucosal ulceration of the rectal area is common in homosexual males.[6]

The prevalence of colitis and rectal lesions among homosexuals is such that they may mask the symptoms of intestinal lesions resulting from Kaposi's sarcoma.[7]

The trauma of sodomy also produces a unique

A brief, less clinical work, written by a physician for laymen, is *Gay Men's Health: A Guide to the AID Syndrome and Other Sexually Transmitted Diseases,* by Jeanne Kassler (Harper and Row, 1983).

form of inflammatory psoriasis in previously unaffected areas. This psoriasis extends from the rectum to the pubic area, penis and scrotum. This is known as Kobner's phenomenon.[8] During sexual activity, the thin silvery scales which have formed on the inflamed areas are rubbed off, leaving the skin raw, bleeding and exposed to infection. The friction against existing hemorrhoids also leaves their surface vulnerable.

Written before the discovery of HTLV–III/LAV as the AIDS agent, a national case study found:

> Blood from rectal mucosal lesions [which] are known to be common in homosexual males who engage in rectal intercourse, could contain the infectious agent responsible for this epidemic.[9]

It is interesting to note that this important study detailing the correlation between homosexual behavior/diseases and the prevalence of AIDS was published by the American College of Physicians in August of 1983. There has only been occasional mention of the relationship between homosexual acts/diseases and AIDS transmission in the national media or press. Usually it is in the context of stressing the susceptibility of heterosexuals through IV drug abuse. One major article doing reasonable justice to this correlation was finally published in the December 1985 issue of *Discover*. However, it unwisely downplays the potential of heterosexual transmission of AIDS.

The damage to the rectal wall facilitates access to the bloodstream of AIDS-infected sperm and other disease-causing organisms. Anal receptive sodomy has been definitely linked to AIDS transmission. In studying the depressed immune systems of practicing male homosexuals in New York City it was found that

> receptive anal intercourse was the specific sexual activity which correlated most strongly with reduced levels of helper T-cells [resulting in immune dysregulation].[10]

DANGERS TO THE ACTIVE PARTNER

The opening of the urethra, along with penile abrasions and lesions resulting from sexual activity and disease, permit infected bloody secretions seeping out of the damaged rectal tissues to enter the bloodstream of the active partner.

DANGERS TO OTHERS

The weakening of the sphincter through repeated sodomy results in fecal incontinence and the dribbling of blood-stained contaminated stool. The involuntary depositing of AIDS virus infected fecal secretions on the benches in locker rooms, toilet seats and elsewhere also creates a potential for spread by this route.

HOW SODOMY SUPPRESSES THE IMMUNE SYSTEM— EVEN WITHOUT AIDS

Sodomy has proven debilitating to the immune systems of passive recipients apart from AIDS infection.[11] During sodomy, the naturally aggressive properties of sperm combined with damage to the rectal wall enable spermatozoa to penetrate the mucosal lining.

A report in the April 27, 1984, issue of *Science* by researchers at the Department of Obstetrics and Gynecology, Cornell Medical Center, New York, stated that occurrence of AIDS among homosexuals

> may have some relation to circulating antibodies evoked as a result of semen deposition in the alimentary canal [intestine]. Human seminal fluid apparently contains components that potentially can suppress the immune response.[12]

A few weeks later other researchers reported in *Lancet:*

> A homosexual individual is repeatedly exposed to viral antigens such as herpes and sperm antigens which can be absorbed through the intact intestine or through mucosal lesions. [*Note:* Bleeding lesions are not necessary for absorption of spermatozoa and harmful infectious agents during sodomy, but they do facilitate it.]
> Host immune responses can be modified by exposure to sperm, with the subsequent formation of anti-sperm antibodies[13] [emphasis added].

During normal heterosexual intercourse, the dynamic qualities of sperm enable penetration and fertilization of the female ovum, resulting in impregnation. The walls of the vagina are elastic and several layers thick, and they have glands which provide natural lubrication during sexual relations. This prevents large quantities of sperm from entering the bloodstream.

A 1984 study in the *Journal of the American Medical Association* noted that the association of sperm-induced immune dysregulation with the practice of anal intercourse

> underscores the critical structural differences between the rectum and the vagina. While the lining of the vaginal mucosa comprises a squamous multilayer epithelium capable of protecting against any abrasive effect

during intercourse, the lining of the rectum is made of a single layer of columnar epithelium. The latter, unlike the vaginal epithelium, is not only incapable of protecting against any abrasive effect, but also promotes the absorption of an array of sperm antigens, thus enhancing their exposure to the immune apparatus in the lymphatic and blood circulation. The high immunogenicity possessed by spermatozoa, coupled with the microbiological flora of the rectum, can work in synergism to generate a state of chronic antigenic stimulation.

In this connection, four of seven immunodeficient female sexual partners of male patients with acquired immune deficiency syndrome (AIDS) also engaged in anal intercourse. An analogous phenomenon can be extracted from the strong association between the high frequency of seroconversion for hepatitis B virus and the routine practice of "passive" anal-genital intercourse.[14]

During sodomy, the biological design of the rectum combined with the aggressive properties of sperm expedite their substantial entrance into the bloodstream. When this occurs repeatedly, antibodies to sperm develop which circulate and impair the immune system.[15] This happens both apart from and along with infection by the AIDS virus. It likely is a co-factor in HTLV–III infection.

In addition to suppressing the immune system per se, the introduction of sperm containing the AIDS agent has been cited as providing a "Trojan horse" mechanism for the transmission of the HTLV–III/LAV lentivirus:

Leukocytes in the seminal fluid [also present in colitis-induced diarrhea] carried the AIDS virus directly to the lymphoid organs of homosexual partners, thus achieving a highly efficient transfer of the infection to most lymphoid cells.[16]

"MONOGAMOUS" SODOMY IS NOT A SAFE ALTERNATIVE

In a revealing study involving *monogamously* paired homosexual males, three-fourths of the passive partners manifested sperm-induced immune dysregulation.[17] Rectal insemination also alters immune responses in rabbits.[18]

The immune dysregulation induced by sperm appears to debilitate the system quite apart from infection by the AIDS virus. Although AIDS development per se must involve the transmission of the HTLV–III/LAV lentivirus, Mavligit et al. propose that the development of sperm-induced immune dysregulation may "predispose the anal-sperm-recipient homosexual males to the more severe phenomena of opportunistic infections and Kaposi's sarcoma."[19]

Sonnabend et al. assert that

immune responses to semen may provide a background of immune suppression, not only promoting repeated CMV infection, but also exacerbating the resulting immunologic disorders.[20]

J. J. Goedert et al. state that their research suggests "HTLV–III is sexually transmitted and that the rectal mucosa may be unusually vulnerable to passage of the AIDS agent."[21] From a purely biological perspective sodomy, even apart from the transmission of AIDS, is an intrinsically unsanitary and pathological act. In addition, the practice of sodomy has been a primary reason why AIDS has been so readily transmitted and fostered among homosexuals.

Oral-penile copulation is also a frequently employed form of homosexual gratification.[22] Infected semen received into the mouth provides a source of infection through abrasions or lesions on the gums, tongue and or roof of the mouth.

Venereal diseases affecting the mouth and throat are especially problematic among homosexuals. Often going unrecognized for a period of time, the resulting lesions provide ports of entry and exit for the AIDS virus. AIDS-infected saliva also is a potential danger involved in oral copulation.

Studies have yet to determine whether or not the gastric juices in the stomach prevent absorption of the potent AIDS virus into the bloodstream after being ingested. Since the eating of AIDS-infected meat is a possible factor in the spread of AIDS among humans, consumption of infected semen may also play a role in transmission.

Other Medical Factors Involved

SADOMASOCHISTIC (S & M) ACTIVITIES
AND THE SPREAD OF AIDS

Activities involving severe bodily abuse and personal degradation are an integral part of the repertoire of homosexual behavior. The damaging practice of sodomy by itself can be classified as a sadomasochistic act. The bloodletting and exchange of contaminated secretions involved in other traumatic homosexual acts further facilitate the spread of AIDS and other diseases. A brief overview of these follows:

MANUAL/ANAL INTERCOURSE—"FISTING"

This practice involves the insertion of the hand, fist and forearm into the rectum and lower colon. In the jargon of participants, it is called "fisting". Fisting causes bleeding lacerations of the intestine and tearing of the sphincter muscle. These internal wounds provide enormous opportunity for the entrance and spread of AIDS virus and other infections.[23] Fisting has been cited as a contributing factor in AIDS cases.[24]

Mechanical devices, dildos, vibrators etc. inserted during fisting have punctured the intestinal wall causing dangerous seepage of fecal matter into the abdomen. If surgery is not performed promptly enough, this can result in death.

In some cases, the damage from fisting is so extensive that a sphincterectomy or colostomy must be performed. Some individuals have then had sodomy performed through the colostomy opening, causing further damage.[25] In San Francisco, where a certain percentage of the murders reportedly are linked to homosexual sadomasochism, a workshop has been offered for instructing homosexuals in how to engage in sex torture without killing each other.[26]

BONDAGE AND DISCIPLINE

Acts in which a dominant partner ties up and tortures the submissive "slave" are also part of the homosexual sadomasochism scene. Those involved are voluntarily bound in painfully tight leather or rubber apparel, whipped, violently sodomized and beaten. Lighted cigarettes are used to burn sensitive parts of the body, especially the genitals, causing ulcers of the penis.[27]

Urination into the mouth and over the bleeding body

of the participant ("golden showers", "water sports") is also a common practice.

Since urine contains the infectious agents for a number of various diseases including AIDS virus infection, this type of behavior is both unhygienic and hazardous. The sores and blisters left on the sex organs also facilitate the entrance of infectious agents into the bloodstream.

"Water sports" are also generally engaged in apart from brutal sadomasochistic behavior. Perhaps that is why a recent "safe sex" guideline from the Gay Men's Health Center published in the October 21–27, 1985, issue of the homosexual tabloid *New York Native* reassuringly advises: " 'Water sports' are considered safe so long as urine does not enter the body."[28]

Some homosexual clubs have slave-auctions in which those who prefer being abused are sold to the highest bidder.[29]

BESTIALITY

Sexual relations with animals has also occurred among a certain segment of the homosexual population. Recently a homosexual club was closed down in New York City where bestiality was one of the practices reported among patrons.

Although citing the need for further epidemiologic and viral studies, Peter K. Lewin, MD, Msc, FRCPC, of the Hospital for Sick Children in Toronto, speculated about the human origin of AIDS being linked to this practice:

> Visna virus is endemic in some flocks of sheep in Europe, where it is called maedi-visna, and causes a neuro-degenerative disease not unlike that seen in the late stages of AIDS in some patients.

Cases of AIDS have been reported from certain urban areas in Northwestern Europe known for their lax sexual mores. One could speculate that a homosexual community in such an area may have become infected by one member's having had sexual contact with a diseased sheep. *Once a homosexual community with international connections has become infected, spread of AIDS becomes inevitable*[30] [emphasis added].

Diseases

The occurrence of AIDS among heterosexuals in Africa has been frequently stressed as proving that the AIDS virus has no special affinity for homosexuals. One medical pundit recently suggested, "The virus has no intrinsic attraction for gays, and gays have no mysterious susceptibility to infection."[31]

What is not being said is that there are a number of diseases and infections common among the African patients with AIDS, especially those with Kaposi's sarcoma, and homosexuals in the United States which are uniquely endemic to both groups but are not generally found among Western heterosexuals.

The African villager at risk for Kaposi's Sarcoma and the homosexual male at risk from AIDS share evidence of past exposure to an identical range of viral and protozoal infections [especially CMV, EBV, HSVI and II, HBV and Entamoeba histolytica].[32]

Among those in developing nations, these disorders are frequently a result of extreme poverty: lack of adequate sanitation resulting in sewage-contaminated food and water supplies and unhealthy living conditions.

Among Western male homosexuals, the prevalence

of these diseases is distinctly related to unhygienic sexual practices which facilitate the spread of infectious agents.

It is true that AIDS has developed in persons who previously had their immune systems intact. It is also true that the rapidity and severity with which the AIDS virus conquers the immune system varies among those infected. When the immune system has been disrupted by certain infections and diseases prior to exposure to HTLV-III, this seems to enhance the destructive effect of the virus.

> T-4 [helper] cells [in the immune system] may be most susceptible to infection when they have been stimulated and their numbers increased by chronic parasitic or viral infections.[33]

Among practicing male homosexuals in the United States, there are a number of grave infections and diseases prior exposure to which has been strongly correlated with the prevalence of AIDS.

Dr. Gordon Muir incisively states, "The real story is that there are several epidemics running loose", not all of them permanently confined to the homosexual subculture.[34]

HEPATITIS B

Hepatitis B virus infection (HBV) is a major cause of acute and chronic hepatitis, cirrhosis and liver cancer.[35] Among practicing male homosexuals in the United States, hepatitis B infection has been pandemic for years prior to AIDS. Homosexual practices, notably sodomy and oral/anal contact, have been key factors. Trauma to the rectum and penis as a result of sodomy and oral lesions from venereal disease provide ports of entry and exit for the virus.

Ostrow writes:

Unlike Hepatitis A infection, fecal-oral spread was not
considered an important route of transmission. Instead,
HBV was thought to be transferred from acute or chronic
carriers to other susceptible persons through shared
toothbrushes, razors, or fomites. Quite the opposite now
appears to be true in homosexual men. Oral-oral transmission may also occur if HBV gains entry through
minute lesions in mucosal surfaces.[36]

"Studies show that between 50 and 75 percent of gay
men have or have had hepatitis B."[37] Writing before the
discovery of HTLV–III, Ostrow noted,

In light of the fact that 90% of homosexually active men
demonstrate chronic or recurrent viral infections with
herpesvirus, cytomegalovirus (CMV) and hepatitis B, it
is possible that these recurrent or chronic infections
may themselves be triggering factors for the development of acquired immunodeficiency.[38]

"In the United States, homosexual men have a higher
prevalence of hepatitis B infection than any other
group."[39] It is estimated that from 5 to 10 percent of
homosexual males are chronic carriers of hepatitis B.
This rate is fifty to one hundred times higher than
the national average of 0.1 percent.[40] Homosexuals
have

... an HBsAg [Hepatitis B surface antigen detectable
in large quantities in serum] positivity rate 40 to 60
times higher than the general population.
Considering the early age at time of infection and the
high attack rates, one might expect *all* sexually active
homosexual men to eventually become infected with
Hepatitis B virus[41] [emphasis added].

Since the routes and prevalence of AIDS transmission bear a striking resemblance to those of hepatitis B,[42] this has enormous implications in terms of the level of AIDS infection in this group as well.

It should also be noted that

rectal mucosal lesions, usually including punctate bleeding points, have been reported to occur in homosexual men with persistent hepatitis B virus infection.[43]

The bleeding lesions induced by hepatitis B also provide ports of entry and exit for the AIDS virus. IV drug abusers also frequently contract hepatitis B through the use of contaminated needles. Their estimated rate of seropositivity is 55 to 65 percent.[44]

An enlightening illustration of the prevalence of hepatitis B infection among high-risk group members is provided by a letter to the editor of the *Lancet:*

Sir, Over a decade SWISSAIR crews will typically spend 300-400 nights in tropical countries, most of which are high risk for viral hepatitis. A perennial question has been—should such personnel regularly receive passive immune prophylaxis or, more recently hepatitis B vaccine? We have studied the risk for hepatitis virus infections in cockpit and cabin staff. . . .

The most outstanding feature [of this study] was that male flight attendants (employees and candidates) significantly more often had anti-HBs and/or anti-HBc antibodies (20-33%) than did either flying personnel (1.4-5.6%) or Swiss blood donors (4-8%).

During the year, 13 of the total of 2664 flying personnel had manifest hepatitis, an incidence of 5 cases per 1000 per year. The estimated incidence of acute hepatitis in the Swiss population is 0.5-0.8 cases per 1000 per year. This high incidence of hepatitis amongst flying personnel was mainly accounted for by male flight attendants, who represent only 19% of all flying personnel but among whom 7 of the 13 hepatitis cases arose. Five cases were of the hepatitis B type (HBsAg positive), and of these 4 occurred amongst the male flight attendants. Thus, the observed high frequency of HBV immunity in male flight attendants was reflected by their high incidence of hepatitis B. Frequent HBV infections in this occupational group probably have little to do with being a flying airline employee—since candidates already showed signs of increased HBV infections. It rather reflects a different HBV exposure due to a life style outside professional duties. Amongst the many explanations, homosexuality might be the most realistic. Worldwide, male cabin attendants are often homosexual, and we have hints that this might not be different in SWISSAIR.

Cockpit personnel and female flight attendants are not at a special risk for HBV or HAV infections, despite exposure in high risk areas, and so they do not need active or passive immunisation against viral hepatitis infection. However, for male cabin attendants, as for other individuals with a high risk life style, active or passive immunisation could be warranted.

A more detailed report will be published in *Aviation, Space, and Environmental Medicine.*

— F. Holdener, SWISSAIR Medical Service, Zurich Airport, Zurich, Switzerland

— P. J. Grob, Section of Clinical Immunology, Department of Medicine, University Hospital, Zurich[45]

DELTA HEPATITIS

On June 7, 1985, the Centers for Disease Control (CDC) stated in their *Morbidity and Mortality Weekly Report:*

The delta virus (also known as hepatitis D virus [HDV]) by some investigators) is a defective virus that may only cause infection in the presence of active HBV infection.

... Infection may occur as either co-infection with hepatitis B or superinfection of a hepatitis B carrier, each of which usually cause an episode of acute hepatitis. Co-infection usually resolves, while superinfection frequently causes chronic delta infection and chronic active hepatitis. *Both types of infection may cause fulminant hepatitis.* ...

Routes of delta transmission appear to be similar to those of hepatitis B. In the United States, delta infection occurs most commonly among persons at high risk of acquiring HBV infections, such as drug addicts and hemophilia patients. ...

Persons who are HBsAg carriers are at risk of delta infection, especially if they participate in activities that put them at high risk of repeated exposure to hepatitis B (*parenteral drug abuse, homosexuality*). However, at present there are no products available that might prevent delta infection in HBsAg carriers either before or after exposure [emphasis added].

A study discussing "Fulminant Delta Hepatitis in Chronic Hepatitis B Infection" was presented in the November 16, 1984, issue of the *Journal of the American Medical Association:*

Case 1: A 36-year-old homosexual man was hospitalized with a two-week history of malaise and a two-day history of weakness and jaundice. He had become confused on the day of admission. He had been using IV drugs for ten years. ...

On examination, he was jaundiced and disoriented in time, person and place. He had numerous spider angiomas over the upper part of the chest and back. ...

Fulminant hepatitis was diagnosed, and the patient was treated along conventional lines. Despite intensive support, deeper coma and renal [kidney] failure developed, and he died on the tenth hospital day. ...

Case 2: A 28-year-old Filipino homosexual man had had malaise of two weeks' duration and nausea, vomiting and jaundice since four days before admission. He had been living in the United States for 11 years and denied IV drug use, but admitted to having multiple sexual partners. He had previously received treatment for syphilis as well as for three episodes of gonorrhea.

On admission, he was alert, well oriented and jaundiced. There were no stigmata of chronic liver disease, and the liver and spleen were not palpable. . . .

On the fourth day of admission, he became confused and belligerent, and coma developed shortly thereafter. Despite intensive care, his condition steadily deteriorated and he died on the ninth day after admission.

The researchers stated that the delta agent appeared to have a role in producing fulminant hepatic failure in each of the cases. They commented:

The impressive clinical course in these two patients emphasizes that superinfection with delta agent is a major potential complication of chronic infection with hepatitis B. . . .

There is a potential danger of acute delta infection spreading in areas where hepatitis B infection is endemic. This has recently been observed in Venezuela, with a high incidence of fulminant hepatic failure. It is noteworthy that our second patient was a homosexual who did not use IV drugs. It has been emphasized that delta infection is particularly associated with an Italian background, IV drug use, and multiple transfusions, but *we have recently been observing delta infection in non-drug-abusing homosexuals*[46] [emphasis added].

INTESTINAL PARASITES AND HEPATITIS A: "THE GAY BOWEL SYNDROME"

"The gay bowel syndrome" was a term used as far back as 1976 to describe the prevalence of a group of rare bowel diseases, previously considered "tropical", among male homosexuals in the United States.[47]

The main conditions considered to be part of this syndrome are:

Amebiasis: a disease of the colon caused by parasites (*Entamoeba histolytica*). Causes dysentery and sometimes liver abscesses. Can result in diffuse inflammation and ulceration of the distal colon that can be mistaken for Crohn's colitis. Usually picked up from contaminated food.

Giardiasis: a parasitic (cause: *Giardia lamblia*) bowel disease causing diarrhea. Can result in severe enteritis (inflammation of the intestinal tract), producing symptoms ranging from acute diarrhea to chronic malabsorption. Spread in similar way to amebiasis.

Shigellosis: a bacterial bowel disease which can cause severe dysentery. In children it can be fatal. Contaminated food is the usual cause.

Hepatitis A: a viral liver disease spread by fecal contamination, e.g., food, water and close person-to-person contact.[48] Dr. Oscar Felsenfeld, in *The Epidemiology of Tropical Diseases,* notes:

> Infectious hepatitis is transmitted in the same manner as other intestinal infections, namely, by water, food, hands and fomites [surfaces] contaminated with feces from an infected person. Experiments on human volunteers have shown that minute amounts of feces are able to transmit the infection.

In describing an outbreak of hepatitis A at a boarding school he states:

... not only were foodhandlers thought to have propagated the disease but also the water that splashed on the seats of the toilets was implicated.[49]

In developing nations, such as various areas in Africa, these diseases are prevalent because of poor sanitary conditions such as sewage-contaminated food and water supplies. They are also readily transmitted by infected food handlers.

Among male homosexuals, these diseases are rampant because of oral-anal practices involving the ingestion of fecal matter.[50] In a type of oral-anal intercourse, the tongue is inserted directly into the rectum (anilingus, "rimming"), and the infected, parasite-laden secretions and fecal matter are swallowed. The practice of outright defecation/ingestion is also involved. In homosexual slang, this practice is commonly referred to as "scat", derived from the French word for feces. Fecal contamination of the fingers during sexual activity is also a means of spreading these diseases.

It is estimated that 30 to 50 percent of practicing homosexual males have contracted parasitic amebiasis as a direct result of these and other practices involving fecal contamination.[51] Dr. Hunter Handsfield, director of the Sexually Transmitted Disease Control Program, Seattle-King County Department of Health and Dr. Anne Rompalo report:

> Sexual transmission of amebiasis was initially suggested in reports of cutaneous amebiasis of the penis and perianal area. Subsequently both amebiasis and giardiasis have been found to be epidemic in homosexual men, and in New York City E. histolytica, G. lamblia, or both are found in up to 40% of homosexual men attending STD [sexually transmitted disease] clinics. Similar prevalence figures have been reported in San Francisco, Seattle,

and Cleveland. . . . Anilingus is believed to be the major mode of transmission.[52]

Dr. Claire Panosian and Dr. Sherwood Gorbach of the Department of Medicine, Division of Infectious Diseases, Tufts-New England Medical Center, Boston, Massachusetts, write:

> With the emergence of highly visible urban homosexual communities during the past decade, bathhouses and clubs where multiple, often anonymous, sexual contacts are sanctioned have gained increasing popularity. This commercial mode of sexual access clearly enhances the uncontrolled circulation of intestinal pathogens in male homosexuals. Even without contact tracing to verify a venereal route of exposure, convincing evidence of heightened transmission is found in the rising incidence of several intestinal infections among adult males in cities such as San Francisco and New York. We have gathered comparative board of health data on the isolation of Shigella from 15- to 45-year-old male cohorts in several major cities to illustrate this trend further [including New York, Los Angeles, Seattle and Boston].
>
> Although the increment in transmission may be largely ascribed to the homosexual community, the potential for wider dissemination also obtains. As Dritz has written of the San Francisco experience, "In 1979 . . . an average of 10% of all patients and asymptomatic contacts reported to the San Francisco Department of Public Health because of positive fecal samples or cultures for ameba, Giardia and Shigella infections were employed as food handlers in public establishments."
>
> . . . In addition, half the homosexual men in Seattle with shigellosis reported recent sexual contacts in other cities such as San Francisco, Los Angeles, Vancouver, and New York, suggesting that intercity spread must be

considered in this infection as with other sexually transmitted diseases (STDs).

They conclude:

> From the time of Moses there has been concomitant
> consciousness of the benefits to the public health of
> careful fecal disposal. Although man's technical ingenu-
> ity has achieved remarkable strides in the purification
> of our immediate domestic environment, the recent
> increase in transmission of intestinal infections among
> homosexual males offers new challenges in preventive
> medicine for physicians caring for these patients.[53]*

The occurrence of AIDS among this group has also
been found to be associated with exposure to feces
during sex and past treatment for enteric (intestinal)
parasites.[54]

In addition to the spread of intestinal parasites, the
ingestion of infected, blood-stained fecal matter may be
a source of AIDS transmission among this group. Sexual contact involving feces has been cited as a factor in
AIDS transmission. In one bathhouse situation, there
was an outbreak of parasites among the patrons through
the shared usage of an enema nozzle used for rectal
douching.[55]

Dr. Donald Abrams of the AIDS KS Clinic, San
Francisco, California, and Dr. Richard Pearce in a letter to *Lancet* on AIDS and parasitism state:

> Sir, Your May 12 editorial on the cause of AIDS (acquired
> immunodeficiency syndrome) mentions several co-factors

---

*As evidence of early sanitation procedures, the physicians cite
Deuteronomy 23:12, 13 which states: "Designate a place outside
the camp where you can go to relieve yourself. As part of your
equipment have something to dig with, and when you relieve yourself,
dig a hole and cover your excrement" (NIV).

that may predispose to infection with human lymph-otropic retrovirus type III (HTLV–III). Omitted, how-ever, is parasitism. As Dr. Rene and colleagues report (April 21, p. 915), homosexual men, Haitians, and Zairians with AIDS share common non-opportunistic intestinal parasites. They ask whether a combination of such intestinal infections could "favor the development of AIDS".

It may be significant in this regard that Japanese researchers have found an association between parasite infection and HTLV–I serpositivity among inhabitants of Okinawa and the Goto Islands. Patients with AIDS from three of the known risk groups (homosexual men, Haitians, sub-Saharan Africans) and monkeys with sim-ian AIDS have been reported to harbour or have a history of exposure to one or both of the parasites *Entamoeba histolytica* and *Giardia lamblia.*

Semen, one of the co-factors mentioned in your editorial, may also contribute to immune alterations in the homosexual risk group. Common to all risk groups is exposure to other foreign antigens (e.g., factor VIII, blood cells or platelets), or endogenous immunosup-pression (e.g., pregnancy), which when coupled with HTLV–III, may result in fulminant AIDS.[56]

VENEREAL DISEASES

Practicing homosexuals are beset with a host of vene-real diseases often occurring simultaneously.

Syphilis: Over 50 percent of reported cases of syphi-lis in the United States occur in homosexual men. Pri-mary syphilis in this group commonly occurs in the rectal area.[57] A history of syphilis has been associated with development of AIDS.[58]

Incurable genital herpes: This incurable disease is almost ubiquitous among practicing male homosexuals.

Infections can occur concurrently in the rectum, penis and mouth. Among homosexuals, infection with herpes has been associated with squamous cancer of the tongue and cancer of the rectum.[59] It has also been associated with nasopharyngeal cancer, cancer of the cervix and Burkitt's lymphoma.

In addition, herpes-type viruses have been shown to suppress specifically T-lymphocyte function aimed at recognizing and mounting an immune response toward the viral antigens.[60]

Perianal herpes virus infection and herpes proctitis are common in homosexual men. In the acquired immunodeficiency syndrome, some patients seem especially predisposed to more intractable and progressive forms of this infection.[61]

Cytomegalovirus (CMV): CMV is found in semen, and the repeated exposure of the rectal mucosa to the virus has resulted in high frequency of CMV infections among homosexuals.

Asymptomatic shedding of virus in urine and particularly in semen facilitates sexual transmission of this pathogen. Intense and repeated exposure of homosexual men to infected secretions containing high titres of cytomegalovirus could contribute to immunodepression and Kaposi's sarcoma [a cancer of AIDS] in this population.[62]

Available data strongly suggest the involvement of CMV in Kaposi's sarcoma.[63]

Venereal warts: Anal warts are a common disorder among practicing male homosexuals.[64] They cause intense itching, and produce a fetid discharge which is highly offensive to others and embarrassing to the sufferer.[65] They are highly resistant to treatment. These warts appear in large cauliflower-like masses in and around the anus in addition to infecting the penis. Anal coitus and elimination of the stool become excruciating and result in further rectal trauma. Various homosexual periodicals contain numerous advertisements by physicians offering specialized treatment for these and other related maladies.

Some of the diseases mentioned above appear to suppress immune function prior to exposure to the AIDS virus. Others, with their recurring sores and lesions, provide ports of entry which facilitate transmission of the AIDS virus.

Both male and female prostitutes are also frequently afflicted with various simultaneous venereal diseases because of their high number of sexual partners.

As the AIDS virus suppresses the immune system, preexisting infections like CMV and herpes run amok through the body. CMV may invade the heart, lungs and other vital organs. Large blackened herpetic boils, up to several inches in diameter, can form across the mouth and rectum.[66] Fulminant herpes is one of the most gruesome aspects of progressive AIDS infection. Entire sections of the face can be rendered unrecognizable by the explosive, bloody hemorrhaging of the skin.[67]

From a biological perspective, therefore, there are several objective reasons why homosexual acts per se have proven to be such an effective means of transmitting AIDS and other debilitating diseases.

1. Sodomy, fisting, the use of mechanical devices and other practices produce tears, fissures and lacerations of the rectum. This trauma facilitates the entrance of infected sperm and pathogenic organisms into the bloodstream.

2. Infected bloody secretions leaking through the damaged walls of the rectum transmit the disease to the active partner through the urethral opening and through open sores and abrasions of the penis produced as a result of bodily abuse and disease. Fellatio, manual-genital and anal-oral sexual practices involving the ingestion of infected semen, blood-streaked fecal matter and secretions facilitate transmission of pathogens.

3. Incessant, oftentimes simultaneous sperm-induced immune dysregulation, liver damage, intestinal parasites and venereal diseases all abet debilitation of the immune system prior to and along with infection by the AIDS virus.

Defining acts such as sodomy, fisting, anilingus etc., as being unnatural is not a matter of homophobic prejudice. Empirical medical evidence clearly demonstrates that the rectum is not designed for intromission of actual or makeshift sex organs, fists, forearms and the like.

Social Factors Abetting
AIDS Spread among Homosexuals

One of the most important lessons I've learned is that there is no such thing as a "decent interval" that must pass before you may enjoy sex again or begin a new love, both of which help you to heal. . . . Four months after Bobbi died, my new roommate moved in.[68]

The social behavior patterns of male homosexuals/ bisexuals have also been a major causative factor in the aggressive and rapid growth of AIDS and other virulent diseases. Sexual interaction in the homosexual community has been characterized by extremely high rates of random, promiscuous and oftentimes anonymous involvement.

In their comprehensive work *Homosexualities,* Bell and Weinberg, both advocates of homosexual liberation, reported that the majority of homosexual males have scores of sexual partners in a year. Over a brief period, this encompasses hundreds of encounters. Over a lifetime, it may involve thousands.[69]

The advent of the homosexual liberation movement dates from the Stonewall Riot on Christopher Street in New York City on June 27, 1969. For decades past, the police department there had a policy of cracking down on the homosexual bars and clubs which were promoting homosexual activity. Raids on establishments fostering homosexual activities were frequent. Public toilets which were being cruised by homosexuals for anonymous sexual encounters were subject to inspections by the vice squad. Those caught engaging in homosexual activities were arrested and prosecuted. Bathhouses designed for mass homosexual encounters were usually clandestine, few in number and subject to constant threat of being closed down.

On June 27, 1969, the Police Department raided an after-hours homosexual bar. The patrons rioted, throwing bottles and bricks at the officers conducting the raid. From that time forward, the homosexual liberation movement flourished with a rapidity and militancy that had not been seen in the annals of Western civilization. The slogan, "Out of the closets and into the streets!" became the battle cry of the movement.

Concurrent with the outspoken militancy among homosexuals, there came a lessening of legislative restraints against pornography, sodomy and establishments fostering homosexual activity.

Homosexual liberation organizations and student groups sprang up rapidly around the country. Colleges and schools which attempted to bar such groups were overruled by the courts. Homosexual bars, clubs and bathhouses burgeoned as the centuries-old legal and societal proscriptions against homosexuality were overturned.

Clubs and bathhouses in particular have come under severe criticism as the number of AIDS casualties have multiplied. Although frequently advertisements for these bathhouses describe the body-building apparatus, saunas and other trappings of a neighborhood health club,

> the baths, despite the services they provide (steam rooms, whirlpool baths . . . etc.), exist primarily to facilitate impersonal sexual encounters among homosexual men. The major function of the bath is to provide an inexpensive place where homosexual men can engage in frequent, anonymous sexual activities without fear of social or legal reprisal. . . . [While there] a patron might have nearly a dozen sexual encounters. . . . [70]

Upon entering, patrons undress and lie about exposed in positions which indicate the type of homosexual acts they wish to engage in.

Along with providing a hub of social interaction, many of the homosexual bars also maintain rooms for patrons to engage in individual and group sex. Homosexual movie houses and peep shows also facilitate anonymous sexual interaction among the patrons. In a recent study in Houston, Texas, 11 percent of the cases of syphilis reported at a clinic were traced back to anonymous sex taking place at peep shows.[71]

A *New York Times* investigative report noted that homosexual clubs have dimly-lit orgy rooms specifically designed to facilitate anonymous, mass homosexual encounters.[72] In the more avant-garde establishments, sadomasochism and bestiality are part of the activities.

For those desiring the quintessential in depersonalized sex, there is a unique contrivance known in underground argot as the "glory hole". This is an aperture in the partition between private booths in the baths, peep shows and public toilets (discreetly known as "tearooms") which permits total sexual anonymity.

In his carefully documented treatise *The Homosexual Network, Private Lives and Public Policy* Enrique Rueda comments:

> The degree of promiscuity in the baths defies the imagination of those not familiar with homosexuality. From the point of view of traditional values, they are probably some of the most destructive and degrading institutions in America today.... From the medical point of view, the baths constitute a major focus for the transmission of disease. Psychologically, they constitute the antithesis of mental health. Ethically, it is difficult to justify the impersonality and degradation they institutionalize.[73]

Supporting these conclusions is the 1983 study in the *Annals of Internal Medicine* in which homosexuals diagnosed with full-blown AIDS admitted that 50 percent of their previous sexual partners, averaging several score annually, had been in bathhouse/club encounters.[74]

The response of homosexual activists to calls for shutting the bathhouses has generally been hostile and defensive. Many fear that legislative action initially aimed at prohibiting the activities there could lead to further restrictive measures. Reinstatement of anti-sodomy statutes, mass quarantine and discrimination in hiring and housing are seen as undesirable potential ramifications.

Only a few of these clubs and bathhouses have actually been shut down by public authorities. In some areas, the courts have ordered them reopened in response to protests by homosexual activists. Although a decline in attendance has been reported by public health officials, the owners of these establishments report that if they were not making money they would be closing their doors voluntarily.[75]

The media and some public health officials maintain that homosexual males in the United States and elsewhere have overwhelmingly positively responded to the AIDS crisis by making drastic alterations in their behavior patterns. The ostensible widespread adoption of so-called "safe sex techniques" and "serial monogamy" have been cited as support.

HOPES FOR BEHAVIORAL CHANGE THROUGH EDUCATION

In the meantime, the AIDS epidemic and companion epidemics rage on. Over the past several years, members of the group at primary risk for developing AIDS have been inundated in their publications with leaflets, posters and articles graphically detailing means of reducing AIDS spread. These repeated attempts at enlightenment have proven spectacularly unsuccessful.

For many, changing long established behavior patterns has not been a viable option. The May 1985 issue of the *American Journal of Public Health* presented a study of AIDS and sexual behavior reported by a cross section of homosexuals in San Francisco. The results reveal a grim fatalism about the risk of contracting AIDS:

> A full 92–96% asserted they were still not taking the most basic prophylactic measures to reduce transmission and exposure to AIDS infection. The majority also felt that they had taken all precautions necessary to protect themselves.
>
> 35% of those who agreed that reducing their number of partners would reduce their risk of AIDS had sex with more than five partners the month prior to the sampling.
>
> 69% of the men having three or more sexual partners the previous month agreed with the statement, "It is hard to change my sexual behavior because being gay means doing what I want sexually."[76]

The consequences of this recalcitrance have been severe. In a follow-up study of a segment of 6,875 homosexual men initially seen at a San Francisco City Clinic between 1978 and 1980, the number of those testing positive for AIDS infection increased dramatically from a modest 4.5 percent in 1978 to an epidemic level of 74.5 percent in 1985.[77] The number of those developing pre-AIDS (ARC) and those with full-blown AIDS also increased.[78]

By the end of 1985, Dr. James Slaff, Medical Investigator at the National Institutes of Health, estimated that between 70 and 90 percent of practicing homosexuals in San Francisco and New York City were infected with the AIDS virus.[79]

These results correlate strongly with the percentage of homosexual men (75 to 90 percent) who have contracted hepatitis B. This illustrates the parallels in prevalence and routes of transmission with AIDS virus infection.

A decline in the rates of rectal gonorrhea has been cited as an indication of radical alterations in behavior patterns among homosexuals. Unfortunately, the apparent decline in this type of venereal disease does not correspond with the fact that AIDS infection has risen astronomically in this group over the same period.

In addition, "reducing the number of sexual partners" cannot really be viewed as an effective preventive against acquiring AIDS. AIDS infection in the homosexual population has reached such pandemic levels that according to Dr. James Curran of the CDC, even with substantial changes in behavior the risk of exposure to the AIDS virus would be diminished only slightly.[80]

The contention that the awareness of the danger of AIDS has produced a drastic change in homosexual behavior patterns is also contradicted by the vast number of bars and clubs remaining open. National and regional homosexual periodicals aggressively advertise these facilities as well as cruises, resort areas and apartment houses designed to encourage homosexual encounters. The "Personal" sections of these periodicals contain numerous graphic solicitations for partners to engage in high-risk homosexual activity. Homosexual "escort services" and "masseurs" also ply their trade in these publications. Some of the bathhouses, in an attempt to solicit the patronage of more youthful clientele, offer them special low-priced locker rates. The price of a locker includes full participation in all the activities available.

Thousands of homosexual bars and hundreds of clubs

and bathhouses remain open and in active use throughout the United States. Occasional attempts at closure by local authorities have been met with vehement protests from patrons, civil libertarians and owners of the establishments at risk.

In summary, there is a combination of factors which has served to make practicing male homosexuals prime candidates for rapidly acquiring and widely disseminating AIDS and other virulent diseases.

1. Physiologically damaging sexual practices have facilitated transmission of the infectious agents.
2. Prior stimulation and suppression of the immune system as a result of sodomy and repeated venereal disease appear to increase susceptibility to devastation by the AIDS virus.
3. The aggressive growth of the homosexual liberation movement, combined with legislative sanction of homosexual behavior and meeting places, have fostered extremely high levels of anonymous, multiple-partner sexual encounters.

In a 1983 study done prior to the discovery of HTLV-III, researchers postulated:

> Any hypothesis regarding the genesis of AIDS must explain the recent emergence of the syndrome. The question is "Why now?" We propose that an unprecedented level of promiscuity has developed during the past decade in large urban areas . . . [and] has exposed a subset of men to the immunosuppressive impact of sperm and CMV. *Similar acquired immunodeficiency disorders may become more common because of changing sexual practises.* . . . [81] [emphasis added].

Although the HTLV-III/LAV lentivirus has now been found to be the etiologic AIDS agent, the overwhelming prior and ongoing medical morbidity of the homosexual subculture appears to have provided the ideally suited host milieu for fomenting and spreading AIDS virus infection on a vast scale.

CHAPTER THREE

AIDS SPREAD INTO THE GENERAL POPULATION: THE TIME BOMB IS TICKING

There is a steaming locomotive roaring down the tracks at the general population.[1]
— Mr. Mel Rosen, Gay Men's Health Crisis, New York City, 1983.

AIDS in Central Africa: A Prototype of Worldwide Disaster

Dr. William Haseltine of Harvard Medical School testified before a Senate subcommittee that more than ten million persons are presently infected with the AIDS virus in Africa.[2] The situation there has reached such catastrophic proportions that some governments have begun censoring the flow of information regarding the spread of the disease. Twenty-one of the African countries known to have AIDS epidemics do not report cases to the World Health Organization.[3]

In June of 1984, researchers from the Pasteur Institute, including Dr. Luc Montagnier, reported isolating the AIDS virus from a married couple in Zaire. The husband was diagnosed with full-blown AIDS and his wife with pre-AIDS. In the discussion of the case they comment:

There is strong evidence that AIDS is endemic in central and equatorial Africa. The report of Kaposi's sar-

67

coma in Zambia with clinical and biological findings similar to AIDS and the likely underestimation of cryptococcosis in Zaire are further evidence. . . .

We cannot establish whether they [the couple cited] acquired the AIDS causative agent through sexual relations or independently by other modes of transmission. However, heterosexual transmission is seldom seen in non-Africans. The African AIDS risk category is special because of the unknown mode of transmission of the disease and its endemic pattern in Africa.[4]

A recent report from several groups, including Dr. Gallo's at the National Cancer Institute, indicates that 15.5 percent of an unselected sample of apparently healthy blood donors in Rwanda tested positive for HTLV–III infection. Another group of forty healthy Africans—mainly from Zaire—were found to have an HTLV–III infection rate of 12.5 percent.[5] Another study of Zairians by Dr. Luc Montagnier and others indicated that 5 to 23 percent of a control group tested positive for LAV. Interestingly, the 23 percent figure was among patients hospitalized with tuberculosis or malaria (vide infra).[6]

The investigators in the first study cited believe that the 12.5 percent infection rate with HTLV–III is probably indicative of the prevalence of AIDS virus infection among heterosexual Central African people living in Zairian and Rwandese urban centers. These findings suggest further that AIDS virus infection has spread extensively into the general population in some Central African countries.

HOMOSEXUALITY AND KAPOSI'S SARCOMA

In the United States the ratio of male to female AIDS cases is 14:1. Ninety percent of all AIDS patients in the U.S. diagnosed with Kaposi's sarcoma (KS) have been male homosexuals. In African countries, Kaposi's sarcoma also has a high ratio of males to females. In Uganda, the ratio is 13:1; in Tanzania 14:1; overall, in African reported series the male to female ratio is 10:1. Though not readily admitted by government authorities, homosexuality has been implicated in the high incidence of Kaposi's sarcoma among African males.[7]

> Johns Hopkins professor of medicine Frank Polk cautions against assuming that AIDS in Africa is only spread through heterosexual contact. He recently returned from a research trip to Central Africa, and he believes that homosexuality is more common there than officials care to admit. "It is simply far more repressed, and most often is seen as bisexuality."[8]

CONTAMINATED NEEDLES AND AIDS SPREAD

In Central and Equatorial Africa, however, it is apparent that AIDS has reached pandemic levels among members of both sexes.[9] The use and reuse of contaminated needles in certain tribal customs and in medical facilities with limited supplies has been cited as a factor.[10]

Heterosexual promiscuity has been cited as a significant means of AIDS transmission in several Central African countries.[11] Heterosexuals developing AIDS in Africa through sexual relations have a high incidence of prior infection with venereal disease similar to Western male homosexuals. A high rate of prior or present infection with hepatitis B has also been noted among both groups.[12] Genital ulcerations have a high frequency among AIDS-infected heterosexual males cited in cases in which the disease is believed to have been transmitted heterosexually in Africa. Many of the females infected with AIDS through sexual transmission have been prostitutes. Twenty-five percent of the patients in a study in Zaire had severe mucocutaneous herpes in the anogenital area, indicating anal sex was also a factor.[13]

Almost all patients in a study done in Rwanda were in the middle or upper socioeconomic class. They worked in the private or public sector in urban areas. Researchers reported:

> An association of an urban environment, a relatively high income and heterosexual promiscuity . . . and contacts with prostitutes . . . could be a risk factor for African AIDS.[14]

According to a report of AIDS occurrence in Zaire,

> The situation in Central Africa represents a new epidemiological setting for this worldwide disease—that of significant transmission in a large heterosexual population.[15]

CLOSE PERSON TO PERSON CONTACT

Dr. John Seale has pointed out that both hepatitis B and the AIDS virus are readily transmitted on multi-use, nonsterile needles. In addition,

> they are also easily transmitted by the close, non-sexual contact between cuts, sores and abrasions, and the blood or serum of other people, which commonly occur (particularly in children) in the crowded and unsanitary conditions in which most people on earth live.[16]

In developing countries, many people are beset with a host of ailments leaving open sores and wounds. Sanitary disposal of infected human waste is frequently not performed, resulting in contamination of food and water supplies. Medical facilities are extremely limited, and extensive treatment is not feasible or too costly for most people. Persons in the end-stage of virulent infectious diseases remain at home in regular close contact with others. The ability for contagion to spread rapidly in this type of situation is considerable.

INSECT TRANSMISSION

Mosquito transmission has been implicated in AIDS spread among heterosexuals in Africa.

> Burkitt's lymphoma [a cancer of the lymph glands] is most common in areas constituting a band across Africa, the "lymphoma belt". By strange coincidence, the "lymphoma belt", 15 degrees north and south of the equator, encompasses the areas where Kaposi's sarcoma is endemic.[17]

Dr. Frederick Siegal, a central figure in AIDS research in New York City, commented on the implications of this phenomenon in 1983:

> Insect vectors, such as mosquitoes and flies, play an important role in the spread of disease in Africa and other tropical regions. . . . *The geographical distribution of Burkitt's lymphoma [cancer of the lymph nodes] within equatorial Africa has always been related to hotspots of malaria, transmitted by Anopheles mosquitoes.* To a lesser extent, *the map of Kaposi's sarcoma incidence also reflects this distribution,* although higher altitudes apparently favor that disease over Burkitt's. A reasonable conclusion drawn from these demographic data is that strains of Anopheline mosquitoes, which carry malaria, are somehow involved in the development of

the lymphatic tumor. *Perhaps the role of these insects is actually to transmit the AIDS agent in Africa.* By altering immunity in persons already carrying Epstein-Barr virus or cytomegalovirus (both highly prevalent in Africa), such an agent could lead to the development of Burkitt's lymphoma or Kaposi's sarcoma in those individuals not promptly killed by opportunistic infections[18] [emphasis added].

In a February 16, 1985 report in *Lancet,* researchers studying the differences between the older "classical" type of Kaposi's sarcoma and the new, exceptionally virulent form related to AIDS reported:

> There is little evidence for homosexual activity among African AIDS patients and seropositive subjects. In Africa HTLV–III appears to be transmitted through heterosexual contact or exposure to blood *through insect bites* or scarification. . . .
> Despite the differences in clinical presentation, the two forms of Kaposi's sarcoma seen in Africa may have the same underlying aetiology. HTLV-III infection may act primarily by inducing a degree of immunosuppression that allows Kaposi's Sarcoma, possibly caused by a separate agent, to develop with the atypical, aggressive course, as in transplant recipients who have been chemically immunosuppressed. By analogy, Epstein-Barr-virus-positive lymphomas occur most frequently in regions of *holoendemic malaria infestation* and in immunosuppressed transplant patients[19] [emphasis added].

On September 9, 1985, a combined team of researchers from the unit for Environmental Epidemiology, National Cancer Institute (Bethesda, Maryland), the Laboratory of Tumor Cell Biology, National Cancer Institute, the Institute of Tropical Medicine (Antwerp), and University of Antwerp, and others reported:

A serological survey of 250 outpatients in rural Zaire showed that the prevalence of antibody against HTLV-I, HTLV-II and HTLV-III [the AIDS virus], as detected by enzyme-linked immunosorbent assay [ELISA—the AIDS blood screening test], correlated strongly with level of antibodies against Plasmodium falciparum [the agent for malaria]. . . .

Among other possible explanations for this correlation, the researchers affirmed:

. . . The human retroviruses could be transmitted by mosquitoes or within the parasite itself. Intraparasite transmission of a retrovirus has been suggested by electron microscopic studies of Sparganum proliferum, a parasite of cows.[20]

This implies that the AIDS virus may genetically incorporate itself into the insects at risk so that their subsequent offspring would become carriers of the virus. Insect transmission of AIDS virus infection, therefore, may not necessitate mechanical transmission from person to person.

Dr. James Slaff, Medical Investigator at the National Institutes of Health, bluntly avers: "There is epidemiological evidence both in America and in Africa that mosquitoes have the potential to transmit the [AIDS] virus."[21]

Now, most recently, comes a report from Venezuela indicating the presence of HTLV-III virus in a high percentage of a small number of patients studied with acute malaria—25 percent with P. falciparum malaria, 41 percent P. vivax malaria.[22]

Spread of the epidemic has become so overwhelming throughout all strata of the population in various parts of Africa that it may never be possible to determine accurately the early primary routes of AIDS spread. What is known is that right now, through a variety of avenues, there is a lethal pandemic of AIDS spreading throughout the crowded cities and villages of developing nations on a magnitude unparalleled in human history.[23] The situation in Central Africa indicates very strongly that the potential for spread of the epidemic throughout the general population in the Western world is enormous.

AIDS Spread into the General Population in the United States

Although the majority of those diagnosed with AIDS in the United States have been homosexuals, the disease has affected other segments of the population. It is clear that the AIDS epidemic has broken out of its previous epidemiologic closet of confinement. AIDS infection is being disseminated through a variety of means among the general population.

DRUG ABUSE

Among homosexuals, amyl, butyl and isobutyl nitrites, commonly known as "poppers", and other so-called recreational drugs have been commonly used as aphrodisiacs to enable prolonged and magnified sexual arousal.[24] Use of "poppers" has been associated with impaired immune response.[25] Intravenous drug abuse has also been a serious problem. Drug-addicted male homosexuals who shared contaminated hypodermic needles with heterosexual addicts introduced AIDS into this segment of the population.

As of July 26, 1983, 159 (33 percent) of the 485 IV drug abusers with AIDS in the United States were homosexual or bisexual men.[26] AIDS then spread en masse throughout larger numbers of heterosexual IV drug abusers. The sharing of contaminated needles has proved a dangerously effective means of spreading AIDS on a massive scale.

Intravenous drug abusers, primarily heroin addicts, have been the next largest group (17 percent of the cases) developing the syndrome. Research indicates that over 85 percent of the nation's urban drug-addicted population is now infected with the virus.[27]

The rapid onset of the syndrome among persons in this group has been abetted by two major factors. First, prior stimulation and suppression of the immune system appears to predispose many individuals to rapid development of the syndrome.[28] Heroin addiction is a debilitating habit. Sickness, bodily abuse and malnutrition commonly result. In a study by the Veterans Administration, 50 to 65 percent of heroin addicts had prior infection with hepatitis B; many are chronic hepatitis B carriers.[29]

Second, repeated direct injection of the virus into the bloodstream through the sharing of contaminated needles greatly increases the number of exposures and facilitates access of the AIDS virus to vulnerable cells.

AIDS-TAINTED BLOOD SUPPLIES—A TRAGEDY THAT COULD HAVE BEEN LARGELY AVOIDED

Although scarcely mentioned, it was well known in medical circles for years prior to the onset of the AIDS epidemic that hemophiliacs and others receiving blood transfusions had been contracting hepatitis B and hepatitis non-A, non-B at an enormous rate. It was also well established that hepatitis B infection had reached pandemic proportions among male homosexuals years before the onset of the AIDS epidemic.

> Little concern has been expressed about the long-term complications of liver disease associated with haemophilia. . . . The prevalence of abnormal liver function tests in haemophiliacs increased rapidly with the widespread introduction of factor VIII and IX concentrates in the mid-1970s. *These abnormalities are believed to arise as a sequel to viral infection transmitted by blood products.* . . . Although few reports of death attributable to liver disease in haemophilia have appeared, we predict that this will become more common[30] [emphasis added].

Delta hepatitis, which has made grave inroads among homosexuals, has also become an increasing problem among blood recipients.[31]

Dr. Gordon Muir has pointed out:

> The question, usually met with thundering silence, is why was it only in 1983, after the AIDS scare, that homosexuals were discouraged from giving blood?[32]

Even then, the CDC advisory that homosexuals not involved in a stable relationship ought to refrain from donating blood was not issued until March of 1983, nine months after they reported the first cases of AIDS among hemophiliacs.

BLOOD TERRORISM AND THE
AIDS BLOOD SCREENING TEST

Robert Schwab, a homosexual activist dying of AIDS and late president of the Texas Human Rights Foundation, asserted:

> There has come the idea that if research money [for AIDS] is not forthcoming at a certain level by a certain date, all gay males should give blood . . . whatever action is required to get national attention is valid. If that includes blood terrorism, so be it.[33]

Shortly thereafter, the AIDS blood screening test was developed to prevent the continued contamination of the blood supply by high-risk group members infected with AIDS. The test, which has been widely hailed as the solution for continued donation of AIDS-tainted blood, has a major flaw: it still permits a significant number of persons who are asymptomatically carrying the virus to slip through. Dr. Roslyn Yomtovian writes in the *New England Journal of Medicine* of February 7, 1986:

> . . . There are now published case reports of individuals who are HTLV–III viral culture positive, but HTLV–III antibody negative. The frequency of such cases is currently unknown. Such persons may be nonresponders to the specific inciting antigens or produce levels of antibody below the technical level of detectability. . . . Because data on HTLV–III test sensitivity are lacking or incomplete, all we can conclude is that the blood is now safer than it was before, but just how safe is unknown.[34]

In Australia, it has been reported that homosexuals as a group were donating blood at a rate 300 percent higher than the general population.[35]

The uproar over false positives has been a red herring from the start. All blood initially testing positive goes through a painstakingly accurate triple-stage screening process which eliminated this problem from the start. This includes the enzyme linked immunosorbent assay (ELISA), Western blot and immunofluorescence assay. Dr. Robert Gallo, commenting on the claims by some medical spokesmen in New York that no one really knows what a positive AIDS blood test means, stated categorically that when the entire series of tests are run, a positive result will be a true positive indicator of AIDS virus infection in 999 out of 1000 cases.[36] Dr. James Slaff comments:

> Another favorite semantic game played by advocates of "moderation" is the claim that "we do not really know the significance of seropositivity" (i.e., a positive blood test for the AIDS virus). That is also ridiculous. If the blood test is performed rigorously, and if an initial positive outcome is confirmed by another test (e.g., Western blot), we *do* know the significance of seropositivity. In 999 out of 1,000 cases, it means that the individual has been infected with the AIDS virus! Infected individuals should consider themselves to be infectious [capable of infecting others] for an undetermined amount of time; they should refrain from sex, postpone marriage and not bear children. . . . They may at any time, without warning, develop AIDS or ARC.[37]

The response of some in the medical establishment for a ban of homosexuals from donating blood was negative. Dr. Selma Dritz, San Francisco's assistant health director, asserted: "Flatly ruling out blood donations from an entire segment of society would be defamatory."[38]

Researchers from the American Red Cross National Headquarters reported in the August 8, 1985, *New*

England Journal of Medicine that 83 percent of AIDS-tainted blood screened out by the ELISA test was donated by admitted homosexual or bisexual males.[39]

In March 1985, physicians in England also reported:

> The acquired immune deficiency syndrome (AIDS) occurs most commonly in homosexual men. This group carries the greatest risk of transmitting AIDS by blood transfusion.... A leaflet describing the importance of AIDS and listing high risk groups was prepared by the Department of Health and Social Security; it implied that only promiscuous homosexuals should voluntarily exclude themselves from giving blood. Subsequently the leaflet was revised to state that this advice applied also to non-promiscuous male homosexuals.
>
> Despite the leaflet, at our transfusion centre some male homosexuals still gave blood....
>
> Donors in the high risk category said that they had continued to donate despite the publicity about AIDS because the original (unrevised) leaflet had implied that homosexuals with stable relationships were still eligible as donors....
>
> It is alarming that some male homosexuals still donate blood, and it is vital that all possible measures are taken to discourage this.[40]

It is estimated that virtually all hemophiliacs in the United States and elsewhere who have received clotting factor concentrates derived from blood collected in the United States prior to 1985 have become infected with the AIDS virus.[41] Nine thousand hemophiliacs plus an additional twenty thousand other blood transfusion recipients are now permanently infected with the AIDS virus.[42] Many, if not most, will die of full-blown AIDS or subsequent brain disease. Many of their spouses and children will also die.[43] There is now a dramatic upswing in transfusion-related cases of full-blown AIDS. This will increase as the virus incubates due to the present large number of those already infected.

Hemophiliacs and other victims of HTLV–III tainted blood have been used by the media to support the contention that AIDS is not particularly related to homosexuality. Hard evidence reveals that the vast majority of hemophiliacs and other blood recipients have fallen prey to liver disease and AIDS infection as a direct consequence of blood donated by homosexuals.

The contamination of the nation's blood supplies with AIDS is a problem which could largely have been avoided if the medical establishment had appropriately restricted male homosexuals from donating blood years before the AIDS epidemic began, as they had good reason to do. As it stands now, persons knowingly at risk for AIDS who donate blood still are not subject to any legal penalties. Since some persons infected with AIDS are able to pass the test undetected, the blood supply still cannot be described as safe.

In the July 4, 1985, issue of the *New England Journal of Medicine,* researchers from the Food and Drug Administration, the Centers for Disease Control and Biotech Research laboratories reported on samples of blood collected during the month of October 1984. This was eighteen months after blood-collecting facilities had begun special screening procedures relating to AIDS, including specific requests for members of groups at increased risk for AIDS to exclude themselves voluntarily from donating blood. They reported:

It is also clear that even though special screening procedures of donors for AIDS had been in place for 18 months before these samples were collected, persons with HTLV–III antibody and virus were still donating blood.[44]

Dr. James Curran of the CDC states equivocally:

Although donations by persons at risk for AIDS may always have been lower and have *probably* declined since 1983, *it is reasonable to assume that guide-lines alone will not totally prevent donation by these persons*[45] [emphasis added].

Heterosexual Intercourse and AIDS Spread

In the United States heterosexual sexual transmission has comprised only a fraction of diagnosed AIDS cases. Only one percent of all AIDS cases have been linked directly to heterosexual relations. An additional six percent involve persons with no known risk factor.[46] Some of these cases may involve heterosexual relations. These percentages have remained relatively constant since the onset of the epidemic.

The remarkably smaller proportion of diagnosed AIDS cases occurring through heterosexual relations may be due to a variety of factors.

1. *Less vulnerable nature of heterosexual intercourse.* Normal heterosexual coitus is not an intrinsically damaging act as is sodomy. Heterosexual acts per se do not result in the bloodletting that is common in homosexual behavior. The anatomical differences between the vagina and the rectum appear to be largely responsible for the fact that AIDS may be acquired more readily by anal-receptive sodomy.[47]

Heterosexual drug addicts who repeatedly inject themselves with AIDS-tainted needles have proved highly susceptible to developing AIDS.

2. *Lack of prior immune suppression.* Some researchers believe that the existence of co-factors, such as sperm-induced immune dysregulation, prior infections with venereal disease, intestinal parasites etc., have a triggering effect which sets off active replication by the AIDS virus.[48] Dr. Jeffrey Laurence, an AIDS researcher at New York Hospital-Cornell Medical Center, states:

> T-4 cells [the T helper cells instrumental in mounting a defense against invading germs] may be most susceptible to infection when they have been stimulated and their numbers increased by chronic parasitic or viral infections.[49]

Parasitic diseases of the intestine among Western heterosexuals are not nearly as prevalent as they are among Western homosexuals (40 to 50 percent or more) and persons in developing nations.[50]

In the West, the epidemic of hepatitis B, like AIDS, has occurred mostly among homosexuals, drug addicts and recipients of large quantities of blood products. Until the advent of the hepatitis B vaccine, it was also a problem among medical workers.[51] Eighty percent of all high-risk group AIDS patients in the United States have evidence of prior exposure to hepatitis B.[52] In the African cases of heterosexual AIDS, prior or present infection with hepatitis B has also been high.[53]

Among heterosexual drug addicts, the repeated direct injections of the virus into the bloodstream, combined with their previous medical morbidity, also appear to heighten its lethal effects.

3. *Lower levels of sexual interaction among heterosexuals than among homosexuals.* Among homosexuals,

the nature of their acts, combined with the extremely high frequency of homosexual encounters (including ten partners or more at a single bathhouse/club visit), facilitates massive invasion of the AIDS virus into the bloodstream and susceptible cells.

4. *Longer incubation period and different pathogenesis.* Among persons infected with the AIDS lentivirus through heterosexual intercourse, the incubation period may be longer and its pathogenesis or mode of destructive operation different. The lack of preexisting co-factors (hepatitis B, intestinal parasites etc.) among the general heterosexual population may retard the development of severe immune suppression.[54] It may take several years longer for those who are infected with lower quantities of the virus and who are not immunosuppressed prior to infection to develop the syndrome. However, persons who are infected with the virus but do not develop severe immune suppression may be more likely to fall prey to subsequent progressive brain dysfunction. The mean incubation period for AIDS virus-induced dementia has been suggested to be fifteen years.[55]

HETEROSEXUAL TRANSMISSION IS OCCURRING

Although the proportion of reported AIDS cases occurring through heterosexual relations has been small, this may soon change. It is increasingly being recognized that normal heterosexual coitus is not impervious to AIDS transmission.

Among horses, the lentivirus which causes equine infectious anemia is transmitted through copulation, insects and contaminated needles.[56] Apparently ignored by the American medical establishment and media, Dr. Luc Montagnier and other researchers at the Pasteur

Institute presented a lengthy study delineating the similarities between the AIDS virus and the equine infectious anemia virus in 1984.[57] Both are lentiviruses.

In the September 20, 1985, issue of the *Mortality and Morbidity Weekly Report* the CDC states:

> For persons born in the United States, female-to-male sexual transmission of HTLV–III/LAV has been less evident than male-to-female sexual transmission. The reasons for reported differences in the epidemiologic pattern of AIDS infections in the United States and certain developing countries are not clear. However, there are at least two possible explanations for the paucity of reported male "heterosexual contact" AIDS patients in the United States. First, female-to-male transmission of HTLV–III/LAV may be less efficient than male-to-female-transmission. . . . Second, the proportion of women among infected persons is relatively small. . . .
>
> While additional evidence for female-to-male transmission of HTLV–III/LAV in the United States is being sought, it would seem prudent to assume that such transmission occurs. In all other sexually transmitted infections, transmission is bi-directional [male to female and female to male], and HTLV–III appears to be spread bi-directionally in other populations. HTLV–III/LAV has been isolated from semen and presumably, would be present in the menstrual blood and the lymphocytes found in cervical and vaginal secretions of infected women.[58]

Dr. James Curran, Director of AIDS Activity at the Center for Infectious Diseases, states:

> The identification of HTLV–III/LAV in lymphocytes and semen is compatible with heterosexual as well as homosexual transmission.[59]

It is apparent that women who engage in anal copulation with an infected male partner are at high risk of acquiring AIDS. The May 19, 1983, issue of the *New England Journal of Medicine* presented a study of seven female sexual partners of men with AIDS. All the men were drug addicts. One of the women developed the full-blown syndrome and five had ARC. Four of the women had engaged in anal intercourse with their partners. Researchers concluded that their study suggested "subjects who are sexual partners of heterosexual men with AIDS are at risk of acquiring the syndrome".[60]

A study in the March 15, 1985, issue of the *Journal of the American Medical Association* reported that five of the spouses of seven married male patients with AIDS and ARC had evidence of AIDS virus infection. Three of the women also had evidence of ARC. The actual means by which AIDS virus infection was transmitted (e.g., blood or semen to blood; blood or semen to mucous membrane; saliva to mucous membrane) was not determined. Researchers reported that their study suggests:

... the relationship between spouses is an efficient mechanism for transmission of the virus and the disease. *It is therefore evident that heterosexual activity has the potential of playing a significant role in human-to-human transmission of HTLV-III and HTLV-III disease* [*AIDS*][61] [emphasis added].

There is also evidence of female-to-male transmission of AIDS. In an article in the October 18, 1985, issue of the *Journal of the American Medical Association,* heterosexual contact was implicated in fifteen of the forty-one ARC or AIDS cases recognized at Walter Reed Army Medical Center. Nine out of ten of the men infected acquired the disease through heterosexual promiscuity, notably sex involving prostitutes. The researchers commented:

The heterosexual transmission of viruses is well documented. For example, the epidemiology of HTLV–III disease [AIDS] resembles that of hepatitis B virus, an agent clearly heterosexually transmissible....

As suggested in this study, prostitutes were probably exposed to HTLV–III by sexual exposure to HTLV–III infected males, possibly bisexual males or males from endemic areas such as equatorial Africa. Concurrent use of IV drugs could also be a contributing factor in some instances. Prostitutes could serve as a reservoir for HTLV–III infection for heterosexually active individuals....

Although military patients may be particularly reluctant to admit to certain risk behaviors, corroboration of patient information was obtained by interviews with family members and other acquaintances and by physical examination, including a rectal culture for gonorrhea, before including these patients in the heterosexual acquired disease category.

They concluded:

... The demonstration of bidirectional sexual transmission of HTLV–III infection and disease has important ramifications. The ultimate impact that HTLV–III disease [AIDS] will have on the heterosexual community will be dictated by the extent of HTLV–III infection in the community, the natural history of the infection, and the presence or requirement of cofactors that modulate the development of disease. Currently, the extent of ARC and AIDS documented in the heterosexual community is limited; however this is another population that should be considered at risk for both disease acquisition and HTLV–III transmission.[62]

Major Robert R. Redfield, MD, of the Department of Virus Diseases at the Walter Reed Army Institute of

Research, Washington, D.C., commented on the results
of the study:

> I don't know of any virus yet that only goes from
> men to women, so I think it stands to reason we'll
> be seeing more of this transmission from women to
> men.[63]

FEMALE TO MALE TRANSMISSION

Among female prostitutes, the high frequency of sexual
encounters, combined with the exposure to large numbers of anonymous partners (thirty to forty per week is
not uncommon), results in bodily trauma and a high
incidence of venereal disease. The resulting genital
lesions and sores provide ports of entry and exit for the
AIDS virus. These diseases may also provide co-factors
which are believed by some researchers to help trigger
reproduction of the virus and development of the
syndrome.

Data obtained from Africa and here in the United
States indicates that bisexual and heterosexual promiscuity are viable means of spreading AIDS on a vast
scale. In Africa, infected female prostitutes and their
patrons have been cited as major sources of AIDS
transmission. According to a report in the *Kenyan Weekly
Review,* more than half of all female prostitutes tested
in Nairobi, Kenya, have become infected with the AIDS
virus.[64] In the United States, 40 percent of the prostitutes in a small study in Miami, Florida, were found to
be infected with the AIDS virus. Studies indicate that
AIDS infection among female prostitutes is on the rise
in other metropolitan areas.[65]

Millions of American heterosexual males and females

are afflicted with a spectrum of venereal diseases causing lesions and blisters. These also provide ports of
entry and exit for AIDS transmission.

Transmission of the AIDS virus through heterosexual
relations, however, does not require damaged vaginal
tissue, venereal lesions or sores. A report from the
Divisions of Viral Diseases and Host Factors, Center for
Infectious Diseases (CDC), states:

> Direct intravascular [virus to blood, such as occurs in
> sodomy and needle sharing] exposure would certainly
> allow virus adequate access to susceptible lymphocytes.
> Mucous membrane exposure might be less likely to
> result in virus-lymphocyte contact, but our recent suc-
> cess in infecting a chimpanzee via vaginal exposure
> without trauma or coexisting infection shows infection
> can occur readily.[66]

In a 1985 study reported in *Lancet,* four out of eight
women who were artificially inseminated with semen
from a symptomless AIDS carrier became infected with
the AIDS virus. One has already developed pre-AIDS.[67]

Writing in August 1984, Dr. Gordon Muir postulated
that the potential of the AIDS epidemic spreading
through the general population could be related to its
ability to become more virulent in form.

> If the AIDS agent is indeed a virus, a worrisome possibil-
> ity is that changes in virulence will take place, now that
> the disease is in the amplification system of homosexual
> promiscuity. It may be that the AIDS agent underwent
> some change in 1979 that triggered the sudden appear-
> ance of the epidemic. John Maddox [editor of *Nature,* a
> leading scientific journal] asks, "May it [the virus] change
> again, becoming in the process a more generalized infec-
> tion in people?"
> In the microbial world there are precedents. . . . The

result could well be the real "final epidemic", the description given by a group of physicians to the effects of a nuclear exchange between the U.S. and the USSR.[68]

HETEROSEXUAL PROMISCUITY

Whether the outbreak of heterosexually transmitted AIDS in the West is related to an increased virulence of the AIDS lentivirus or other factors such as a more lengthy incubation period in less immunocompromised persons is uncertain. Prior lack of immune suppression, the less vulnerable nature of normal coitus and substantially lower levels of sexual interaction—meaning lesser quantities of the virus invading the body—may have served to make heterosexual transmission less apparent earlier.

Whatever combination of factors may be involved, the present increase in AIDS cases among heterosexuals in the United States could begin to follow the increases among homosexuals of several years ago. The incidence of heterosexual AIDS in the United States can be expected to increase greatly, based on existing trends of heterosexual AIDS infection.

Sexual Terrorism and AIDS Spread

"Every now and then", says Dr. John Dwyer, the former Chief of Immunology at Yale–New Haven Hospital, who has treated more than 400 AIDS patients, "there are people who say, 'I know I'm going to die and I'm going to take as many people with me as I can.' "[69]

Reminiscent of the attitude displayed by Japanese kamikaze pilots during World War II, this sentiment was reflected in the remarks of a homosexual prostitute diagnosed with AIDS in Houston, Texas. He stated publicly that he would go back to plying his trade as soon as he was released from the hospital. Police and public health officials were at a loss as to how to prevent him from disseminating the disease. According to legal regulations, it was necessary to observe him in a high-risk act with a customer before he could be restrained. He later died of AIDS.

In New Haven, Connecticut, a female prostitute with full-blown AIDS was released from a hospital and returned to work as a streetwalker. She presented a threat to the public health, but city officials did not want to invoke quarantine powers. She was finally arrested on prostitution and drug charges and eventually died in jail.[70]

The September 23, 1985, issue of *Time* reported a similar case in Alameda County, California. A male homosexual came down with AIDS and was treated several times at the county public health clinic for gonorrhea. He had sexual relations with three to five partners a week without informing them of his condition. Dr. Robert Benjamin of the county Bureau of Communicable Diseases called him "a sociopath". "There are people like him everywhere", Benjamin said.

Some high-risk group members, while perhaps not deliberately trying to infect others, maintain an insouciant fatalism about contracting or transmitting AIDS that is deeply disturbing to those in the health care field.

While commenting on the fact that private physicians in New York City have been banned under edict of the Health Department from using the AIDS blood screening test in private practice, Dr. Helen Singer Kaplan, the head of the Human Sexuality Program at the New York Hospital-Cornell Medical Center, asserted:

Gays put pressure on the Board of Health to forbid the test. *We would stop the spread of AIDS today if these high-risk people, these typhoid Marys, would stop spreading the disease.* As a physician and a scientist, I'm appalled at their wildly having sex and spreading AIDS[71] [emphasis added].

High-Risk Group Members and the Widespread Dissemination Of AIDS

Upwards of one and a half million homosexual/bisexual men are presently infected with the AIDS virus.[72] Robert Hawkins, associate dean at the School of Allied Health Professions, Health Sciences Center, State University of New York at Stony Brook, reports that most male homosexuals report having had sexual activity with women.[73]

The analysis of homosexuality by Bell and Weinberg indicates that as many as 65 percent or more of practicing homosexuals report having engaged in heterosexual coitus and 20 percent or more are or have been married.[74] This latter figure corresponds to the percentage (18 percent) of homosexual AIDS patients who report having been previously married.[75] Dr. Jay Levy of the University of California School of Medicine and researchers from the School of Public Health, University of California, Berkeley, recently presented a study on the "Potential for Transmission of AIDS-Associated Retrovirus [ARV] from Bisexual Men in San Francisco to Their Female Sexual Contacts". They concluded:

... A possible chain of transmission for ARV infection from homosexual men to women would be through bisexual men. ...

A substantial potential clearly exists for epidemic spread of ARV infection to women in San Francisco. To date, there is no evidence that such extension has occurred. However, ascertaining the possible spread of the epidemic to this population through establishment of a serological surveillance system should be an urgent priority.[76]

It should also be noted that there is a substantial potential for epidemic spread of AIDS infection to women in other areas of the country with large homosexual/bisexual populations.

Dr. William Haseltine of Harvard's Dana-Farber Cancer Institute has reported the following in Congressional testimony regarding the potential for AIDS spread through female prostitutes:

A recent survey completed in West Germany also indicates that the infection of the prostitute population is a problem of major proportions. Nationwide, about twenty percent of all prostitutes in Germany are infected. Infection rates differ widely depending upon whether the prostitute population is registered, operating under license from the government and subject to routine health examination, or whether the population is unregistered. Infectious rates in the registered population are about one percent, whereas the infection rate in the unregistered population, largely drug abusers, ranges between twenty and fifty percent. In one study, more than half of the unregistered prostitutes working the area of Berlin near the train station were found to be infected.

There is accumulating evidence that infection is transmitted from prostitutes to their customers. A recent study conducted by the United States Army revealed that five percent of United States soldiers reporting to venereal disease clinics in Berlin are now infected with the AIDS virus. In the United States one and one half percent of soldiers treated at the venereal disease clinic at Fort Bragg, Georgia, were found to be infected with the AIDS virus. . . . *A lethal venereal disease is now spreading through our population,* all the more dangerous because infections may remain inapparent for a long time[77] [emphasis added].

Upwards of 85 percent of the United States urban drug-addicted population is infected with the AIDS virus as well. Within this group of an estimated 250,000 persons, are thousands of infected women, many of whom support their drug habit through prostitution.

Each of these groups constitutes an enormous reservoir of AIDS infection capable of spreading the epidemic.

CHAPTER FOUR

CASUAL TRANSMISSION—
AN UNDERRATED DANGER?

... Caution is in order when knowledge is incomplete so that the public interest can be protected.
— Dr. Richard Restak

In May of 1983, before the infectious agent for AIDS was discovered, Dr. Anthony Fauci, Director of the National Institute of Allergy and Infectious diseases, remarked:

> If . . . non-sexual, non-blood-borne transmission [of AIDS] is possible, the scope of the syndrome may be enormous.[1]

AIDS Prevention Guidelines for Medical Workers

A year previously, in 1982, the CDC issued precautions for medical workers caring for AIDS or pre-AIDS patients. They included:

1. Extraordinary care must be taken to avoid accidental wounds from sharp instruments contaminated with potentially infectious material and to avoid contact of open skin lesions with material from AIDS patients.
2. Gloves should be worn when handling blood specimens, blood-soiled items, body fluids, excretions, and secretions, as well as surfaces, materials and objects exposed to them.

3. Gowns should be worn when clothing may be soiled with body fluids, blood, secretions or excretions.

4. Hands should be washed after removing gowns and gloves and before leaving the rooms of known or suspected AIDS patients. Hands should also be washed thoroughly and immediately if they become contaminated with blood.

5. Blood and other specimens should be labeled prominently with a special warning, such as "Blood Precautions" or "AIDS Precautions". If the outside of the specimen container is visibly contaminated with blood, it should be cleaned with a disinfectant [such as a 1:10 dilution of 5.25% sodium hypochlorite (household bleach) with water]. All blood specimens should be placed in a second container, such as an impervious bag, for transport. The container or bag should be examined carefully for leaks or cracks.

6. Blood spills should be cleaned up promptly with a disinfectant solution such as sodium hypochlorite (see above).

7. Articles soiled with blood should be placed in an impervious bag prominently labeled "AIDS Precautions" or "Blood Precautions" before being sent for reprocessing or disposal. Alternatively, such contaminated items may be placed in plastic bags of a particular color designated solely for disposal of infectious wastes by the hospital. Disposable items should be incinerated or disposed of in accord with the hospital's policies for disposal of infectious wastes. Reusable items should be reprocessed in accord with hospital policies for hepatitis-B-virus-contaminated items. Lensed instruments should be sterilized after use on AIDS patients.

8. Needles should not be bent after use, but should be promptly placed in a puncture-resistant container

used solely for such disposal. Needles should not be reinserted into their original sheaths before being discarded into the container, since this is a common cause of needle injury.

9. Disposable syringes and needles are preferred. Only needle-locking syringes or one-piece needle-syringe units should be used to aspirate fluid from patients, so that collected fluid can be safely discharged through the needle, if desired. If reusable syringes are employed, they should be decontaminated before reprocessing.

10. A private room is indicated for patients who are too ill to use good hygiene, such as those with profuse diarrhea, fecal incontinence or altered behavior secondary to central nervous system infections.[2]

In the 1985 guidelines for preventing health care workers from becoming infected by patients with AIDS, the CDC repeatedly denies the possibility of nonsexual, nonblood-related means of transmission.

... The kind of nonsexual person-to-person contact that generally occurs among workers or clients in the workplace does not pose a risk for transmission of HTLV-III/ LAV. ... Because AIDS is not transmitted through preparation or servicing of food and beverages, these recommendations state that food-service workers known to be infected with AIDS should not be restricted from work. ...

The advisory affirms infectious AIDS virus has

been isolated from blood, semen, saliva, tears, breast milk, and urine and is likely to be isolated from other body fluids, secretions, and excretions, but epidemiologic evidence has implicated only blood and semen in transmission.[3]

The guidelines for medical workers, however, warn repeatedly that such workers should avoid contact, not only with the blood of AIDS patients, but with "other body fluids" as well. The following are some representative passages:

> When the possibility of exposure to blood or other body fluids exists, routinely recommended precautions should be followed. The anticipated exposure may require gloves alone, as in handling items soiled with blood or equipment contaminated with blood or other body fluids, or may also require gowns, masks, and eye coverings when performing procedures involving more extensive contacts with blood or potentially infective body fluids. . . .
>
> Because of the theoretical risk of salivary transmission . . . during mouth-to-mouth resuscitation, special attention should be given to the use of disposable airway equipment or resuscitation bags and the wearing of gloves when in contact with blood or other body fluids. Resuscitation equipment and devices known or suspected to be contaminated with blood or other body fluids should be used once and disposed of or thoroughly cleaned and disinfected after each use.[4]

One prominent columnist has raised a thought-provoking illustration of the apparent discrepancy between denials of casual transmission and medical practice:

> Well, then, how come they acted as they did in Paris? There you may have read (in the small print) when Rock Hudson was discharged, all the nurses who attended him—and this was in a modern hospital, not a witch doctor's hut—were made to burn their dresses. The patient was fed on paper and plastic plates, with plastic forks and spoons—which were then destroyed.[5]

The Parallel of Hepatitis B Transmission with AIDS

In regard to potential avenues of AIDS spread, the CDC states:

> The epidemiology of HTLV-III/LAV infection is similar to that of hepatitis B virus (HBV) infection.[6]

Although nonsexual close contact among household members has been repeatedly denied as a possible route of AIDS transmission, in the June 7, 1985, CDC recommendations for protection against hepatitis B it is reported that:

> The role of the carrier is central in the epidemiology of HBV transmission. . . .
>
> Carriers and persons with acute infection have highest concentrations of HBV in the blood and other serous fluids; less is present in other body fluids, such as saliva and semen. Transmission [of hepatitis B] occurs via percutaneous [through skin] or permucosal [through mucosal membranes] routes. Infective blood or body fluids can be introduced by contaminated needles or through sexual contact. *Infection can occur in settings of continuous close personal contact, such as in households.* . . .

Several pages later, it is directly confirmed that

> household contacts of HBV carriers are at high risk of acquiring HBV infection[7] [emphasis added].

The Council on Scientific Affairs for the American Medical Association asserts:

> The distribution of AIDS cases in the United States suggests that the syndrome is caused by an infectious agent *with a pattern of transmission similar to that of hepatitis B.* . . . Hepatitis B may be transmitted through

mucosal surfaces, including the mouth and the eye[8] [emphasis added].

AIDS-Virus Transmission in Families

In the February 16, 1985, *Lancet,* researchers reported a cluster of HTLV-III/LAV infection in an African family:

Acquired immunodeficiency syndrome (AIDS) has been reported in infants and children, as has mother-to-infant transmission, suggesting in-utero or perinatal infection. We report a familial cluster of three Rwandese brothers and their parents with T-cell deficiency and carriage of antibodies to HTLV-III/LAV with features suggesting other routes of transmission. . . .

Because the incubation period for AIDS may extend up to several years, in utero or perinatal transmission of HTLV-III/LAV infection cannot be ruled out. However, the fact that in these children symptoms started developing several months to years after birth raises the possibility of horizontal transmission. Since none of the brothers had received blood transfusions before the onset of their disease, other routes of transmission should be considered, such as breastfeeding, and those postulated for transmission of hepatitis B among children in Africa (routine close contact, scarifications, contaminated needles, and blood sucking vectors).

The varying clinical manifestations observed in this familial cluster also suggest that the clinical spectrum of HTLV-III/LAV infection might not be restricted to full-blown AIDS and AIDS-related complex but might extend to subclinical forms and maybe to asymptomatic carrier states, even in children. Large seroepidemiological studies are needed to clarify the exact routes of transmission of HTLV-III/LAV infection in African children.[9]

The August 5, 1985, *Wall Street Journal* states that a study in Zaire indicates that those who live under the same roof with an AIDS sufferer have a 300 percent higher risk of becoming infected than the general population.[10]

In the November 22, 1985, *Journal of the American Medical Association,* after downplaying the potential of casual transmission, Dr. Fauci acknowledges:

There is indirect evidence to suggest that, when a person is frequently exposed to someone who is [AIDS] virus positive, then there is a greater chance of that person getting infected. But that's not definitely been proven.[11]

In the January 10, 1986, issue of the *Journal of the American Medical Association,* researchers from the Center for Infectious Diseases, Centers for Disease Control reported a study on persons living in close contact with hemophiliacs infected with the AIDS virus and those living with hemophiliacs who were not positive for the AIDS antibody. They found:

Antibody-negative, nonhemophilic contacts of AIDS/ARC and of antibody-positive hemophiliacs had *significantly lower* numbers of lymphocytes, T helper lymphocytes, and T suppressor lymphocytes than did contacts of antibody-negative hemophiliacs....

Persons with hemophilia generally have stable home environments. Thus, ever since they were recognized as being at heightened risk of AIDS, there has been concern and speculation concerning AIDS transmissibility to long-term sexual partners and household members of this at-risk population. Transmission patterns have appeared similar to those of hepatitis B virus, a virus for which this AIDS-risk group is also at risk....

The time between HTLV–III/LAV infection and seroconversion is currently unknown.... Signs of immune dysfunction might be indicative of early [AIDS-virus] infection....

While this could reflect an early response to HTLV–III/ LAV infection, we think these results should be interpreted with great caution pending prospective serial evaluation of these households and similar evaluations of other hemophilic households. However, they could be epidemiologically meaningful, in light of a recent report suggesting that some antibody-negative sexual partners of hemophiliacs were themselves virus positive on repeated cultures.... [12]

Hepatitis B Outbreaks Involving Medical and Dental Personnel

In the November 28, 1981, *Lancet,* doctors from the Section of Clinical Immunology, University Hospital, in Zurich reported:

Cluster of Hepatitis B Transmitted by a Physician
    Over a 4 and ½ year period (1973–77) 41 individuals in a village in eastern Switzerland (population 3000) were admitted to hospital because of acute hepatitis B. This hepatitis incidence was much higher than that in surrounding villages and that in the whole country. An epidemiologic survey showed that one of the two general practitioners in the affected village was the source of infection. He had a chronic aggressive hepatitis B surface and e antigens. No new cases of hepatitis B occurred in the village in the 3 years after his death....

Mode of Transmission
    The fact that no new cases of hepatitis B occurred in village B [the town at risk] in three years following the

practitioner's death is further evidence that he was a source of infection.

Of the original 41 patients with hepatitis B, 5 have chronic hepatitis. . . .

Transmission of hepatitis B infection to health care service personnel is not rare in Switzerland and elsewhere; transmission in the opposite direction has only been reported for oral surgeons, a gynaecologist, and an inhalation therapist, but not to our knowledge for general practitioners. The view that transmission of infection from health care personnel to patient is a rare event has been expressed in editorials and in a World Health Organization report, and has been at least partly substantiated by prospective surveys. However, since many fortuitous circumstances must occur before such events are discovered, the incidence of these events may well be underestimated. The fact-finding in the outbreak reported here was facilitated because the outbreak had occurred in a small, non-migrating, and medically well-surveyed population. The findings support the argument that medical personnel should be vaccinated against hepatitis B in countries where hepatitis B virus infections are not rare.[13]

In February of 1985, the Centers for Disease Control (CDC) reported nine cases of hepatitis B occurring among patients of a dentist who had been unknowingly transmitting the disease. Two of the patients died from fulminant hepatitis and one was paralyzed as a result.

The report notes that acquiring hepatitis B is a significant health risk for dental professionals. Although seven outbreaks of hepatitis B traced to dentists or oral surgeons have been reported, the CDC states that this is an infrequent occurrence. For those dentists who remained carriers and returned to work, "wearing gloves was usually successful in preventing further transmission".[14]

On February 21, 1986, researchers from the Hepatitis Branch, Division of Viral Diseases, Center for Infectious Diseases (CDC) presented a report on "Transmission of Hepatitis B with Resultant Restriction of Surgical Practice".

> Five patients developed acute hepatitis B (HB) within four months after major operations by the same obstetric-gynecologic surgeon. Investigation documented that the surgeon was HB surface antigen and HB e antigen positive; all five patients had an HB subtype matching that of the surgeon and no other identifiable risk factors for HB viral infection. . . . The surgeon resumed his surgical practice but *was required to obtain written informed consent from patients, to double glove,* and to employ appropriate surgical techniques to avoid self-injury. Seven months later, acute HB occurred in a patient two months after a cesarean section, resulting in exclusion of the surgeon from major operations[15] [emphasis added].

As yet there have been no reported cases of CDC-defined AIDS occurring as a result of contact with an infected medical worker. A study of one surgeon with AIDS in the United States found that none of his patients had yet contracted full-blown AIDS. However, the modes of AIDS virus transmission are highly similar to hepatitis B transmission. Dr. James Slaff, Medical Investigator at the National Institutes of Health, raises the following question:

> Is it reasonable to restrict workers in health care and food preparation on the basis of infection with the AIDS virus? Most people would not want to be in physical contact with a doctor, nurse, or dentist who is infected with the virus. A dentist, for example, might conceivably have a portal to the bloodstream when a tooth was being removed. The possibility exists for infected saliva or a small finger cut creating an avenue for transmission for the virus. . . .

The possibility of an infected individual having primary patient contact on a regular basis is certainly troubling. It is equally troubling, though, to consider terminating a health care career that takes years of dedication and a large investment[16] [emphasis added].

Just how troubling this issue is may depend on whether you are a patient at risk of acquiring AIDS-virus infection or a health care worker at risk of transmitting the virus. At the very least, it would seem that patients should have the *right to know* whether their dentist, physician or other primary health care worker is an AIDS virus carrier. In the illustration above, the surgeon at risk of transmitting hepatitis B, which generally has less grave consequences than AIDS, was required to obtain written informed consent from his patients before performing surgery.

As it stands now, a surgeon or dentist who knowingly is carrying the AIDS virus or who has full-blown AIDS or ARC can still perform invasive procedures without telling his patients of his condition. In light of the gravity of AIDS virus infection, it would appear more ethical and in the best interests of the patients at risk to allow them to have an informed choice in this regard.

Insect Transmission of Hepatitis B and AIDS

A 1984 study published by the American Society of Tropical Medicine explains the prevalence of hepatitis B infection in Northern Zaire. It states that in addition to other means, factors contributing to the high incidence of hepatitis B infection there include:

1. The common practices of traditional healers using
    scarification of the skin for treatment of all kinds of
    pain. The instrument used for scarification—mostly
    razor blades—are cleaned with water, but never steri-
    lized in any way.
2. The high promiscuity and polygamy. In recent years
    polygamy has been generally advocated and is prac-
    ticed throughout the country.
3. The enormous abundance of blood-sucking arthro-
    pods [insects]. It has been discussed that blood-
    sucking arthropods may transmit hepatitis B infection.
    The fact that malaria is holoendemic throughout the
    region and the spleen index in the population well
    above 75% gives support to this assumption.[17]

These latter findings support the contention of Dr.
Mark Whiteside and Dr. Carolyn MacLeod, researchers
at the Institute of Tropical Medicine in Miami, that
mosquitoes appear to be a vector in an outbreak of AIDS
in the impoverished community of Belle Glade, Florida.

Dr. Martin J. Blaser of the Veterans Administration
Medical Center, Denver, Colorado states:

Kaposi's sarcoma is highly area-specific in equatorial
Africa, and there is a clustering of cases. Hepatitis B is a
good example of a blood-borne disease with multiple
routes of transmission; the hepatitis B virus has been
isolated from hematophagous [blood eating] arthropod
hosts, including bedbugs. . . .
The presence of HTLV–III infection in spouses of
members of high-risk groups suggests sexual transmission,
but although this clearly occurs it may not account for
all such cases of AIDS in close contacts. Because of the
chronic viremia seen after HTLV–III infection and
the rapidly increasing number of persons infected with
HTLV–III . . . endemic vector-borne transmission in the
United States remains a possibility. If a suitable insect

vector for transmitting HTLV–III is present in the United States, then population groups other than those presently implicated may be at risk for infection. *Considering the long incubation period of AIDS and the relatively constant fraction [6%] of AIDS patients not identified as belonging to a high-risk group despite the increasing number of cases, insect-borne and other forms of transmission should be carefully considered*[18] [emphasis added].

Equine infectious anemia, the lentivirus infection afflicting horses, is spread by the transfer of blood from horse to horse.

The mechanisms [of spread] include insect vectors, needles used for inoculations and blood sampling, and tatooing devices; transfer can also occur during copulation and possibly in milk passed to a suckling foal. The disease kills half its victims; once infected an animal remains infectious for life; the virus can be found in all tissues, including the brain. Treatment is impossible, so spread of the disease can be prevented only by slaughtering infected animals. It is interesting that the virus exists in many immunologically different forms, which makes the theoretical task of producing an effective vaccine difficult, if not impossible.[19]

Saliva: A Viable Means of AIDS-Virus Transmission

In a study reported in the October 1984 issue of *Science,* respected Boston hematologist Dr. Jerome Groopman, along with researchers from the National Institutes of Health, found the AIDS virus contained in saliva of persons at risk for AIDS, both those with ARC and those who were asymptomatic. They concluded:

The recovery of HTLV-III from saliva suggests that direct contact with this body fluid should be avoided since saliva ... could facilitate horizontal [person-to-person] transmission.[20]

On January 11, 1985, the CDC stated: "There is a risk of infecting others by ... exposure of others through oral-genital contact or intimate kissing."[21]

Dr. Slaff states:

Because the AIDS virus has been cultured from the saliva of infected individuals, the FDA currently recommends that infected individuals refrain from "French" kissing. This is a reasonable precaution. Dr. Zaki Salahuddin has provided an example in which intimate kissing was the only possible vector of transmission: an elderly infected woman whose only exposure was kissing her AIDS husband, an impotent transfusion recipient.[22]

Dr. Richard Restak, a prominent Washington neurologist who has been studying AIDS as a brain-related disease, asserts:

At this point live AIDS virus has been isolated from blood, semen, serum, saliva, urine and now tears. If the virus exists in these fluids, the better part of wisdom dictates that we assume the possibility that it can also be transmitted by these routes.

It seems reasonable, therefore, that AIDS victims should not donate blood or blood products, should not contribute to semen banks, should not donate tissues or organs to organ banks, should not work as dental or medical technicians, and should probably not be employed as food handlers.[23]

AIDS Virus Transmission
and Contact Lens Fitting

In the February 15, 1986, issue of *Lancet,* researchers
from the Departments of Ophthalmology and Virology
at the University of Finland reported:

> Body fluids from which human T-cell lymphotropic virus
> type III (HTLV-III) have been isolated include tears. To
> find out if HTLV-III could be transmitted to contact
> lenses we studied volunteers known to be positive for
> HTLV-III antibodies.
>
> Five men and one woman aged 29–43 agreed to wear
> high-water contact lenses in an experiment. Three had
> AIDS-related complex and three had AIDS. The lenses
> were fitted in the afternoon and were removed the next
> morning 14–16 hours later. . . .
>
> HTLV-III was isolated from four patients in contact
> lenses or rinsing solution but not in the small quantity of
> tears. High water content lenses of only one manufac-
> turer were used but it is not very likely that such lenses
> differ significantly in their ability to attract HTLV-III or
> cells infected with the virus. *There then is a potential
> risk in contact lens fitting, in cleaning lenses, and in
> tonometry.*[24]

The Lengthy Survival Time of
the AIDS Lentivirus Outside the Body

Dr. James Slaff, Medical Investigator at the National
Institutes of Health, has reported: "Unlike most other
retroviruses, the AIDS virus can survive outside the
body for hours to days."[25]

The September 28, 1985, issue of the British medical
journal *Lancet* contained a study by a team of French

researchers from the Viral Oncology Unit at the Pasteur Institute revealing that the AIDS lentivirus can remain infectious outside the body for up to ten days.

LAV/HTLV–III, the agent causing AIDS, has been isolated from body fluids (blood, semen, saliva, tears). Its isolation in saliva prompted us to investigate the possibility of transmission by saliva, and we have studied the sensitivity of LAV/HTLV-III at room temperature.... The virus used for the infectivity assay ... was left at room temperature for 0, 2, 4, or 7 days in a sealed tube or allowed to dry in a petri dish. After the times indicated in the figure the virus was used to infect stimulated T lymphocytes and viral production was determined in cell-free supernatant by testing for the reverse transcriptase activity twice a week. [The data] shows the unusual stability of HTLV–III at room temperature. No significant difference was found between 0, 2, or 4 days. Only a slight decrease is noted with a delay in the virus production indicating a loss of few infectious particles *after 7 days* at room temperature.

Two petri dishes containing 25,000 cpm equivalent reverse transcriptase of dry virus were kept at room temperature for 4 or 7 days and then resuspended in 0.220 ml water and used to measure the infectivity. As [the data show], *significant numbers of viral particles are then inactivated, but some infectious virus is still present since release of virus was seen on day 10.* This result indicates that *the virus is resistant at room temperature, either in dry form or liquid medium.*

This resistance of LAV at room temperature may explain the appearance of some cases of AIDS cases in non-risk groups. To prevent possible contamination by viral particles in dry or liquid form hygiene should be increased in the general population. Moreover, some more safety precautions should be taken in laboratories and in hospitals and by dentists who use a vacuum pump for saliva aspiration. Indeed, these data strongly support the use of disinfectants found to be effective against the AIDS agent.[26]

Worries over casual transmission have been dismissed as the product of ignorance, paranoia and homophobia. The public has been repeatedly told that the AIDS agent is an extremely frail virus, incapable of living outside the body for any extended period of time. For instance, in the October 7, 1985, issue of *New York Magazine,* the writer of the article "The Last Word on Avoiding AIDS" states "The [AIDS] virus itself is not hardy.... "

The findings of the French researchers—specialists from the Pasteur Institute's elite Viral Oncology Unit, went unmentioned by major public health officials and were virtually blacked out by the media.

Two months after their findings were published in *Lancet,* the *Journal of the American Medical Association* commented in the Medical News section:

> A recent report from the Pasteur Institute in Paris by the investigators who originally isolated the lymphadenopathy virus suggests that the AIDS virus might be pretty tough. The French study finds that virus survives ten days at room temperature even when dried out in a petri dish.[27]

Six months after the Pasteur Institute study was reported, researchers from the laboratory of Tumor Cell Biology, National Institutes of Health and elsewhere reported findings on the stability of concentrated amounts of the AIDS virus:

> In view of the serious consequence of HTLV-III/LAV infection, its stability under clinical and laboratory conditions and its inactivation by commonly utilized inactivating agents and disinfectants are of tremendous importance

to health care workers and laboratory personnel. Here, the results of testing the stability of HTLV–III/LAV under various experimental conditions are reported. . . .

To test the effect of some frequently encountered clinical and laboratory conditions on the infectivity of the HTLV–III (TM), virus diluted in media supplemented with 50% human plasma was dried and incubated at 23 to 27 degrees Centigrade, or incubated in an aqueous state at one of several different temperatures: room temperature (23 to 27 degrees Centigrade), 36 to 37 degrees Centigrade, and 54 to 56 degrees Centigrade for various periods of time. In a dried state, complete inactivation of virus required between three and seven days. . . .

Exposing virus to different temperatures resulted in a reduction of infectious virus corresponding to increasing times of incubation and increasing temperatures. Complete inactivation . . . of infectious virus was seen between 11 and 15 days of exposure at 36 to 37 degrees Centigrade. Infectious virus was still detected after 15 days at room temperature. . . .

Infectious cell-free virus could be recovered from dried material after up to three days at room temperature, and in an aqueous environment (e.g., water), infectious virus survived longer than 15 days at room temperature. Even under the more rigorous heating conditions commonly used to inactivate complement (54 to 56 degrees Centigrade [133 degrees Fahrenheit]), infectious virus was detected three hours after exposure. . . . The stability of HTLV–III at 54 to 56 degrees Centigrade suggests that the inactivation of virus in blood products (e.g., antihemophilia factors) could require more extensive treatment, as has been suggested.[28]

The lack of accurate news coverage regarding this critical information is highly discomfiting. More disturbing still are the recommendations by the French researchers for guarding against AIDS transmission. They give specific safety precautions for medical and dental personnel which clearly intimate that oral transmission of AIDS through saliva is a danger to be reckoned with. They also advise that hygiene should be increased in the general population. The question of who should disinfect whom, how, what and where are left unanswered. For example, when an AIDS virus carrier coughs or sneezes infected secretions into a punch bowl or salad bar, the AIDS virus could remain infectious for quite some time. When a cook or waiter contaminates food with infected saliva or other body fluids—i.e., coughs, sheds infected tears while slicing onions or sustains a cut and contaminates the food with blood—what should be done? Should one spray or wash the contaminated foodstuffs with chemical disinfectant? Or should the hapless patron simply swallow hard and hope for the best?

In any case, it does appear that a lentivirus which remains infectious for ten days or longer in dry form may be not quite as delicate and innocuous outside the body as has been widely rumored.

Infected Child Care Workers and Food Handlers

In 1983, Dr. Frederick Siegal, then Chief of Immunology at Mt. Sinai Medical Center in New York City, and a central figure in AIDS research, explained the unique vulnerability of young children to infectious agents:

> One factor possibly contributing to the development of AIDS in very young children is the immaturity of the newborn's immune system, which makes it extremely susceptible to other infectious diseases like herpes and hepatitis B. Having in effect a normal immune defi-

ciency in the first days or weeks after birth may thus make infants especially vulnerable to an agent causing AIDS[29] [emphasis added].

That same year, Dr. Sidney Finegold, president of the Infectious Disease Society of America, asserted:

> It clearly would be wise to keep certain personnel ... such as immunosuppressed or pregnant individuals from working with AIDS patients. . . . Pregnant women should also avoid contact with AIDS patients because of the risk of infection with cytomegalovirus as well as the risk of AIDS itself. . . . It would seem prudent to ask that AIDS patients not engage in food preparation or handling for others, particularly if they have an intestinal infection.[30]

In July 1984, Dr. Gene M. Shearer of the National Cancer Institute cautioned:

> If an infectious AIDS agent exists and is opportunistic, with the syndrome being expressed only in immune-deficient persons, then infants with *environmental exposure* to the AIDS agent should be very susceptible[31] [emphasis added].

In the *Morbidity and Mortality Weekly Report* the CDC has presented the following information:

> As of December 1, 1985, 217 (1%) of the 15,172 AIDS cases reported to CDC occurred among children under 13 years of age. Sixty percent of these children are known to have died. These 217 cases represent only the more severe manifestations of HTLV-III/LAV infection. *Less severe manifestations, often described as AIDS-related complex (ARC), are not reported to CDC, so the number of children with clinically significant illness attributable to HTLV-III/LAV infection is greater than the reported cases of pediatric AIDS.* In addition, a number

of infected children are probably asymptomatic[32] [emphasis added].

Six percent of the reported infants and children with AIDS have no known risk factor.

Cytomegalovirus (CMV) Infection and AIDS

Cytomegalovirus (CMV) is a viral infection which frequently infects the unborn baby via the placenta. It is a major cause of abnormal fetal development and death.

> An average of 30,000 CMV-infected infants are born annually in the United States. . . .
> Of the infected infants, 10 percent have severe multiple organ system disease which damages the brain, perceptual organs, lungs, liver and blood; in a few instances it results in death soon after delivery. In the survivors, severe debilitating brain damage, blindness, and deafness are common.[33]

CMV has been implicated in 2,700 to 7,600 cases of congenital birth defects annually in the United States.[34]

Cytomegalovirus (CMV) belongs to the herpes virus family. It is transmitted through semen, urine, blood and saliva. AIDS patients are often infected with Pneumocystis Carinii Pneumonia and CMV simultaneously.[35] The coughing and wheezing associated with AIDS-related respiratory complications indicates a danger of transmitting CMV infection through infected saliva and bronchial secretions. Hence the warning about pregnant women avoiding contact with AIDS patients.

It should be remembered that repeated, active CMV infection is also extremely common in homosexual men. "90% of homosexually active men demonstrate chronic or recurrent infections with herpesvirus, cytomegalovirus (CMV) and hepatitis B."[36]

Intestinal (Enteric) Infections and AIDS

Cryptosporidiosis is a significant problem among AIDS patients. It also poses a health threat to other patients whose immune systems are disrupted.[37]

> Cryptosporidiosis is a parasitic infection normally seen in farm animals and not usually seen in humans. However, patients who are immunocompromised may develop this entity, which may produce profound watery diarrhea and can lead to a fatal outcome.[38]

Dr. Donald Abrams studied a large group of patients with lymphadenopathy syndrome (pre-AIDS or ARC) at the Cancer Research Institute of the University of California at San Francisco. A majority of his patients had stool examinations positive for one or more enteric protozoans.[39] Past treatment for enteric parasites was reported by 44 percent of the homosexual AIDS patients described in a National Case-Control Study. This corresponds to the high rate of intestinal parasites found among male homosexuals in urban areas.

As discussed in Chapter Two, intestinal parasites are readily transmitted by infected food handlers. In addition,

> because protozoal cysts remain viable for prolonged times, often measured in days, fomites (surfaces that adhere to and transmit infected material) such as contaminated rectal tubes as well as towels, mats, walls, floors, and other environmental surfaces are also responsible for some disease spread.[40]

The Risk of Acquiring AIDS during Pregnancy

In the February 9, 1985, issue of *Lancet,* it was reported that a young woman developed symptoms of AIDS six months after receiving a contaminated blood transfusion necessitated by severe postpartum bleeding. Doctors reported that the brief time that elapsed between the point of initial transmission and development of the syndrome was short compared to other cases of transfusion-related AIDS.

> This short latency as compared with other series *could have been favoured by the physiological immunosuppression observed during and shortly after pregnancy, since immunosuppression may trigger the clinical expression of AIDS*[41] [emphasis added].

In regards to the increased vulnerability of pregnant women to AIDS infection, they report:

> *Pregnancy is associated with suppression of cell-mediated immunity and increased susceptibility to some infections.* The T-helper to T-suppressor ratio is decreased during normal pregnancy, being lowest in the third trimester, and returns to normal approximately 3 months postpartum. It is not known whether pregnancy increases an infected woman's risk of developing AIDS or ARC, but one study suggests it does. Fifteen infected women who were well at time of delivery were followed an average of 30 months after the births of their children. Five (33%) subsequently developed AIDS; seven (47%) developed AIDS-related conditions; and only three (20%) remained asymptomatic. These results may not apply to all infected women, *but they do suggest an increased likelihood of developing disease when an HTLV-III/LAV infection occurs in association with pregnancy*[42] [emphasis added].

Lentivirus Transmission in Sheep

The most telling indication of the potential for casual transmission of AIDS is the nature of the AIDS agent itself. The AIDS virus is a highly potent lentivirus. Maedi-visna, the form of lentivirus infection appearing in sheep, kills the animals through a deadly form of pneumonia or through gradual but progressive brain disease. Dr. Slaff of the National Institutes of Health affirms that the visna virus is the animal virus closest to the AIDS virus.[43]

Lentivirus infection in sheep involves a means of spread consonant with casual transmission in man. In the 1976 treatise *Slow Virus Diseases of Animals and Man,* P. A. Palsson described the transmissibility of maedi lentivirus among sheep:

> maedi was successfully transmitted to healthy sheep by direct contact between healthy and diseased animals, by contaminating their drinking water with faeces from diseased animals and by injecting material from typically affected lungs and lymph nodes intranasally [into nasal passages] . . . and intravenously. . . .
>
> In advanced stages of maedi the presence of the viral agent can be demonstrated regularly in various organs. Occasionally maedi virus has also been demonstrated in nasal swabs from such sheep. *During the clinical course of [maedi infection] fits of dry coughing are occasionally seen, and thick mucous is often seen in the larger bronchi.*
>
> *Transmission of maedi by the respiratory route as a droplet spread of the infectious agent while animals are in close contact is considered from field experience to be the most likely way the disease is spread naturally* [44] [emphasis added].

Simply put, the lentivirus which causes lethal pneumonia in sheep is spread by coughing. Dr. Blaser of the Veterans Administration Medical Center in Denver has found that "the earliest manifestation of AIDS in persons native to developing countries is frequently tuberculosis." [45] Dr. John Seale comments:

> Pulmonary tuberculosis is often the initial clinical manifestation of infection with LAV (the AIDS virus) in Haiti and Central Africa. Indeed, it was suggested last month in the *Lancet,* that infection with *M tuberculosis hominis* should be included as a manifestation of lesser AIDS or ARC. CDC remains silent on this absolutely fundamental issue.
>
> Pulmonary infection with *M tuberculosis hominis* is characteristically transmitted via respiratory aerosols. If open, cavitating, pulmonary tuberculosis coexists with chronic lymphoid interstitial pneumonitis caused by LAV, it is inevitable that large numbers of infectious LAV virons, as well as tubercle bacilli, will be expelled in aerosols during coughing. LAV spread by the respiratory route would affect men and women equally; spouses and children of index cases would be particularly at risk, as has already been observed in Africa. [46]

An illustration of the phenomenon described by Dr. Seale was reported in the July 18, 1985, issue of *Lancet.* Researchers from France, including two from the Pasteur Institute, reported:

> We recently examined a Haitian woman with the AIDS-related complex in whom LAV [the AIDS virus] was isolated simultaneously from blood and bronchoalveolar lavage fluid. LAV has previously been isolated from peripheral-blood lymphocytes, saliva, semen, lymph nodes, and brain, but in this case it was isolated from pulmonary secretions [lung fluid].

The woman, who had no history of blood transfusion, drug abuse or sexual promiscuity, was diagnosed as having AIDS virus-induced lymphoid interstitial pneumonitis.[47]

Regarding the less-well-known ability of the AIDS virus to infect cells in the lungs, Dr. Seale wrote recently in the *Journal of the Royal Society of Medicine:*

> ... Chronic lymphoid interstitial pneumonitis (CLIP) is such a characteristic feature of paediatric AIDS that CDC, when it redefined AIDS on 28 June 1985, decided to include CLIP. Serological tests for HTLV–III/LAV antibodies had to be positive, but no evidence of opportunistic infections was required for the diagnosis, provided that it occurred in children under the age of thirteen. Evidence now emerging from Central Africa shows that in the later stages of the AIDS epidemic, large numbers of adults as well as children develop CLIP, often in association with pulmonary tuberculosis.
>
> Pulmonary tuberculosis, combined with pulmonary AIDS, would be highly lethal because both the microbes would be coughed into the air, and both remain infectious for more than a week at room temperature.... [48]

The Wall Street Journal, in 1986, presented a report, "Tuberculosis Rise among AIDS Patients Raises Concern about Wider TB Infection", stating:

> Public health officials are keeping a worried watch on a new epidemic: the appearance of tuberculosis in the same groups of people that are at high risk of developing AIDS.
>
> In the past two years, cases of TB, known as the white plague in the 19th century, have been diagnosed among drug addicts in New York City, among young, white male AIDS patients in San Francisco and among Haitians in Miami....

TB in Miami

In Miami, TB cases grew by 38% last year, with the

largest increases among men in the 25-to-44 age group, says Janice Burr, a Dade County health official. The department had earlier noted occurrences of TB among Haitians with AIDS, but a pattern was also emerging of young, white American-born TB victims, she says. The common element among the victims was the presence of AIDS, she adds. . . .

Increase in San Francisco
1 . . . "We're finding that the incidence of TB in AIDS patients is five times that of the regular population of San Francisco", says Gisella Schecter, tuberculosis controller for the city's health department. San Francisco reported a 10% gain in TB cases in 1985. . . .

In about half of the San Francisco cases, TB was diagnosed before AIDS. But the city doesn't know to what extent tuberculosis is occurring among carriers of the AIDS virus who don't have the disease, she says, because California law restricts the use of the AIDS test. . . . [49]

A textbook for medical students, *The Pathogenesis of Infectious Disease,* by Cedric A. Mims, states:

Respiratory Tract
In infections transmitted by the respiratory route, shedding depends on the production of air-borne particles (aerosols) containing microorganisms. These are produced to some extent in the larynx, mouth and throat during speech and normal breathing . . . more pathogenic streptococci, meningococci and other microorganisms are also spread in this way, especially when people are crowded together inside buildings or vehicles. *There is particularly good aerosol formation during singing and it is always dangerous to sing in a choir with patients suffering from pulmonary tuberculosis.* Microorganisms in the mouth, throat, larynx and lungs are expelled to the exterior with much greater efficiency during coughing,

shedding to the exterior is assured when there are increased mucus secretions and the cough reflex is induced. *Tubercle bacilli in the lungs that are carried up to the back of the throat are mostly swallowed and can be detected in stomach washings, but a cough will project bacteria into the air.*

Efficient shedding from the nasal cavity depends on an increase in nasal secretions and on the induction of sneezing. In a sneeze up to 20,000 droplets are produced and during the common cold, for instance, many of them will contain virus particles. The largest droplets (1 mm diameter) fall to the ground after travelling 15 feet or so and the smaller ones evaporate rapidly, depending on their velocity, water content and on the relative humidity. Many have disappeared within a few feet and the rest, including those containing microorganisms, then settle according to size. The smallest, although they fall theoretically at 1-3 feet per hour, in fact stay suspended indefinitely because air is never quite still. Particles of this size are likely to pass the turbinate baffles and reach the lower respiratory tract. If the microorganisms are *hardy,* as in the case of the tubercle bacillus and smallpox virus, people coming into the room later on can be infected[50] [emphasis added].

Time Will Tell

There has been a vigorous effort on the part of many members of the medical and media establishments to convince the public that there is no danger of transmission of AIDS-virus infection through non-sexual, non-blood transfusion related means. Various studies are often cited which do indicate that persons working in close proximity with AIDS patients have not as yet developed full-blown AIDS or antibodies to HTLV–III. These studies may be reassuring to many people. Nevertheless:

> The unequivocal facts that are not denied by those doing research on the AIDS virus, or on the disease itself, are that the virus is a lentivirus, that it will be extremely difficult to produce a vaccine or cure, that infection is permanent and can occur by several routes, and that the spectrum of fatal disease is much wider than the CDC definition of AIDS. Possibilities which fit the nature of the other lentiviruses but which cannot be assessed yet are that infection in utero may be 100 percent effective and fatal, that the overall fatality rate may approach 100 percent, that it will not be possible to make a vaccine, and, finally, that we are all equally at risk. . . .
>
> If, like the other lentiviruses, the AIDS virus can be transferred to ungulates [hoofed mammals], then we must face the fact that it could be spread in cows' milk (just as it is in breast milk), in bronchial secretions transmitted as aerosols by coughing (as is maedi-visna), and, potentially, by insect vectors, if only mechanically (as is equine infectious anemia). (J. F. Grutsch, Jr. and A. D. J. Robertson, "The Coming of AIDS", The *American Spectator* March 1986, pp. 12–15.)

The information contained in this chapter does not prove that casual transmission of AIDS-virus infection is occuring at present or that it will become a significant means of spread of the epidemic in the future. However, the apparent present lack of evidence concerning non-sexual, non-blood transfusion related means of transmission is not a firm guarantee of actual or potential lack of risk. According to Dr. Montagnier of the Pasteur Institute,

> The potential for genetic variation is perhaps the greatest danger in the future of the AIDS epidemic. . . . A fur-

ther change of the virus in its tropism [ability to infect types of cells] and *ways of transmission* cannot be excluded. (L. Montagnier, "Lymphadenopathy-Associated Virus: From Molecular Biology to Pathogenicity", *Ann of Int Med* 1985;103:689-693.)

Dr. Restak points out:

This disease [AIDS] is only partially understood, is presently untreatable, and is invariably fatal. For these reasons alone, caution would seem to be in order when it comes to exposing the public to those suffering from this illness.

In addition, the incubation period is sufficiently lengthy to cast doubt on any proclamations no matter how seemingly authoritative in regard to the transmissibility of the illness: "The virus may be transmitted from an infected person many years before the onset of clinical manifestations", according to Dr. George Lundberg, editor-in-chief of the *Journal of the American Medical Association.* "Latency of many years may occur between transmission, infection and clinically manifest disease." (R. Restak, "Worry about Survival of Society First; Then AIDS Victims' Rights", *Washington Post,* 8 September 1985.)

CHAPTER FIVE

FADING PROSPECTS FOR A CURE OR VACCINE

The word 'cure' is not even in the vocabulary.
— Dr. Michael Gottlieb, UCLA immunologist

For the forseeable future a workable vaccine is a bad bet....
— Dr. James I. Slaff, Medical Investigator, National Institutes of Health

Major Obstacles to AIDS Treatment

Several factors have made attempts at treating AIDS extremely frustrating and futile thus far. HTLV-III is a virus. In a section on antiviral agents, Goodman and Gilman's authoritative textbook *The Pharmacological Basis of Therapeutics* points out:

> The development of compounds useful for the prophylaxis and therapy of viral disease has presented more difficult problems than those encountered in the search for drugs effective in disorders produced by other microorganisms. This is so because, in contrast to most other infectious agents, viruses are obligate intracellular parasites that require the active participation of the metabolic processes of the invaded cell. Thus, agents that may inhibit or cause the death of viruses are also very likely to injure the host cells which harbor them. Although the search for substances that might be of use in the management of viral infections has been long and intensive, very few agents have been found to have clinical applicability.

Indeed, even those have exhibited very narrow activity, limited to one or only a few specific viruses.[1]

Dr. John Beldekas, an AIDS researcher in the Department of Microbiology at the Boston University School of Medicine, explains further:

> By now we are all familiar with the name of the virus LAV/HTLV-III. This is an RNA virus (or retrovirus), not a DNA virus [although it can become incorporated in the DNA]. A virus is a parasite—it lives off its host for all its processes. It invades a host, takes over the machinery of the cell and reproduces to infect another host. This particular virus is a biological mystery. There are growing pieces of evidence indicating that this virus may be changing its surface characteristics as it is transmitted from one individual to another. These small changes may make it impossible to develop an effective vaccine against it.
>
> There is also another major problem—no one has even constructed a vaccine against an RNA virus before, and no one knows if it will be effective.

Other major factors which have impeded efforts to find a cure or vaccine for AIDS include:

1. *The body's natural defenses are incapable of combatting the AIDS virus.* With other diseases, the immune system produces antibodies which attack and kill invading organisms. Vaccines are utilized to raise antibody levels in the bloodstream high enough to kill invading pathogens. In the case of infection with the AIDS virus, the antibodies which develop have little or no capacity to neutralize the effects of the virus. Researchers dare not inject even a minute amount of the AIDS virus into humans as a means of raising antibodies to ward off the disease. A genetically altered AIDS virus which is not believed to be infective but which probably will induce

antibodies has recently been developed. (See H. M. Schmeck Jr., "AIDS Researchers Begin Testing New Version of Smallpox Vaccine", *New York Times,* April 10, 1986.) However, as researchers pointed out almost two years ago:

> In AIDS as well as in AIDS-related lymphadenopathy, retrovirus production continues despite the presence of detectable titers of antibodies to LAV/IDAV or HTLV-III.[2]

2. *There is no cure for AIDS devastation of the immune system.* The opportunistic infections which plague AIDS patients are devastating and difficult to treat per se. Even when they have been somewhat ameliorated, the underlying progressive destruction of the immune system makes it virtually certain that the infections will return.

Although certain agents have reduced the apparent level of viruses, this effect has been only palliative. The AIDS virus "hides" from antiviral agents. HTLV-III incorporates itself into the DNA (genetic material) of infected cells.

> Once infection by a retrovirus occurs, it is likely to be for the lifetime of the person. Integrated viral genes are duplicated with the normal cellular genes so all progeny of the originally infected cell will contain viral genes.[3]

This means that there is no way for antiviral agents to effectively "get at" all of the AIDS viruses being harbored in the body.

> Although effective therapies are available for many of the infections and tumors that occur in patients with AIDS, no therapy exists for the underlying immunodeficiency.[4]

3. *AIDS virus infection of the brain is untreatable.* The AIDS virus invades and replicates within the central nervous system. The virus has crossed over what is known as the "blood brain barrier". This alone creates virtually insurmountable obstacles in treatment. Since the HTLV-III "hides" by incorporating itself into the genetic material, any type of treatment to kill infected cells in the brain would of necessity involve the destruction of masses of brain tissue.

4. *The AIDS virus is continually mutating.* In all lentivirus infections in animals, antigenic drift during the lifetime of an infected animal produces a variety of antigenic strains which infect the same animal. Dr. Myron Essex and other researchers from the Department of Cancer Biology, Harvard School of Public Health state:

> The lack of successful antiviral immunity in the case of persistent infections with HTLV-III/LAV has led to the hypothesis of rapid mutation and antigenic drift. The mutation rate and degree of genomic variation is known to be high for this virus; with other lentiviruses such as the equine infectious anemia agent and visna virus, antigenic drift can occur with a single infected animal.[5]

This also appears to be the case with HTLV-III in man. A report in the *Journal of the American Medical Association* states:

> ... Since the original isolation of the lymphadenopathy virus by Montagnier and his associates at the Pasteur Institute and of HTLV-III by Gallo and his group at the National Institutes of Health, the AIDS virus has been isolated by many laboratories. Gallo estimates that there are now around 200 isolates of the virus.[6]

Dr. Malcolm Martin, chief of the Laboratory of Molecular Microbiology in the Infectious Diseases Institute notes:

> In contrast to other retroviruses, such as HTLV–I and HTLV–II, this virus is very heterogeneous in genomic structure; its five or six genes are very unstable. The data from our laboratory and others suggest that there isn't a single virus entity isolated from a given person. The same person can harbor multiple forms of the virus.[7]

Dr. Seale comments:

> The almost unlimited varieties of antigenic strains of lentiviruses produced by antigenic drift, combined with the inability of antibody produced by the host to eliminate the virus from circulation, have rendered ineffective all attempts to produce vaccines to prevent lentivirus diseases in animals. Effective protection against infection with the AIDS virus using existing vaccination techniques would seem to be theoretically impossible.[8]

5. *Any vaccine developed would be ineffective for those already infected.* There are already over two million people estimated to be infected with the AIDS virus in the United States alone. All persons in this group are permanently capable of spreading the infection to others. By the time any type of agent is developed that is capable of preventing the AIDS virus from invading the immune system and brain after it has entered the body (assuming that it is even possible), it will be too late for the millions more who will have become infected.

CHAPTER SIX

THE SPECTER OF
CONTINUED AIDS SPREAD

We must be prepared to anticipate that the vast majority of those now infected will ultimately, over a period of 5 to 10 years, develop life-threatening illness.
— Dr. William Haseltine, leading AIDS researcher, Harvard Medical School (*New York Times,* September 27, 1985)

How Bad Is the Problem Right Now?—
Current Sobering Facts

At present, over 25,000 Americans have developed full-blown AIDS. This number will have more than doubled a year from now. An additional 125,000 to 250,000 are suffering with pre-AIDS (ARC). This figure will also double within a year.

Tragically, these figures represent only a fraction of the total number of persons who are presently infected with the AIDS virus. On the basis of CDC surveillance data as of July 1985, physicians at New York Medical College estimated the number of persons infected with the AIDS virus to be much greater than those diagnosed with CDC-defined AIDS. Writing in a 1985 issue of the *New England Journal of Medicine,* they have broken down the estimated number of persons infected with the AIDS virus into the following categories.[1]

ESTIMATED NUMBER OF PERSONS INFECTED WITH AIDS

Homosexuals and bisexuals	1,345,500
Intravenous drug users	270,000
Hemophiliacs	8,970
Recipients of blood or blood products	20,700
Haitians	41,700
Heterosexual contacts of persons	14,400
Persons at no known risk	64,200
Total	1,765,470

Based on current data, as many as 20 percent or more of those presently infected will go on to develop full-blown AIDS. This means that 350,000 new cases of full-blown AIDS will occur over the next several years.

Some 20 to 25 percent of those presently infected, an additional 350,000 to 400,000 persons, will languish with debilitating pre-AIDS (ARC). Along with other grave illnesses besetting persons in this stage, many will suffer from AIDS-induced dementia.

In the next several years, close to one million persons, mostly between the ages of twenty and forty-nine, will have their physical and mental health inexorably and progressively devastated by AIDS virus infection.

Hundreds of thousands—perhaps more—will die of full-blown AIDS. Hundreds of thousands—perhaps more—will suffer from the severe immunological and neurological disorders induced by the HTLV–III virus.

In addition to the loss of human life, the first 10,000 cases of AIDS averaged a direct medical cost of $147,000 per patient. Total economic losses approximated 6.3 billion dollars.[2]

At present cost levels the wave of 350,000 new full-blown AIDS patient could result in an additional 51 billion dollars in direct medical outlays alone [$147,000 × 350,000]. Total economic losses will rise to over 220 billion dollars.

The Catastrophic Consequences of Continued AIDS Spread

If effective steps are not rapidly undertaken to prevent the continuing dissemination of the AIDS virus, the ramifications will not merely be disastrous; they will be catastrophic. If the present growth trend of AIDS infection is allowed to continue unimpeded, the following consequences can be expected:

1. *Massive increase in the number of people harboring AIDS-virus infection.* According to Dr. Dana Bolognesi of Duke University and other experts, the number of those infected with the AIDS virus is doubling annually. Even if everyone of those presently infected formed an exclusively "monogamous" sexual relationship with only one other uninfected individual, the number of those infected would still likely double. Present estimates indicate between two and three million Americans are infected with the AIDS virus. This means an infection level surpassing four million persons by the end of 1986. Looking ahead, this would result in:

8,000,000 by the end of 1987
16,000,000 by the end of 1988
32,000,000 by the end of 1989
64,000,000 by the end of 1990

Even if the present estimated rate of AIDS virus transmission was cut in half (50 percent of those presently and subsequently infected became celibate), that means three million Americans infected with the AIDS virus by the end of 1986, and

4,500,000 by the end of 1987
6,750,000 by the end of 1988
10,125,000 by the end of 1989
15,187,500 by the end of 1990

The latter projections are optimistic. The capacity for an incurable sexually transmitted disease to penetrate vast numbers of the population is fearsome. More than twenty million Americans are already infected with incurable genital herpes, and the rate of those newly acquiring the disease is growing by 500,000 cases annually. This is occurring with a disease that has visible signs (blisters, lesions) and troublesome symptoms between periods of remission. In contrast, persons infected with the AIDS virus can have few signs or symptoms (or none) for an extended length of time.

Barring effective steps being taken to prevent continued transmission, it is conservatively estimated that at least fifteen million Americans will be permanently infected with the AIDS virus by the end of 1990.

2. *Massive AIDS death.* Fifteen million persons infected with the AIDS virus would suggest that at least three million persons will develop and die from full-blown AIDS. This is more than the American casualties suffered in both world wars, Korea and Vietnam combined, concentrated within a single decade.[3]

Forty percent or more of those with full-blown AIDS may be expected to develop severe neurological complications as a result of their disease.[4] These would result from neurological opportunistic infections and/or direct attack by the AIDS virus on brain tissue.[5]

3. *Massive levels of intermediate AIDS, including debilitating illnesses and dementia.* One third or more of the fifteen million persons infected with the AIDS virus will develop AIDS related complex (ARC). As mentioned in Chapter One, the gravity of this secondary stage of AIDS infection should not be minimized. In addition to a host of debilitating illnesses, ARC patients are frequently beset with severe psychiatric disturbances (psychoses, hallucinations, mutism), resulting from AIDS virus destruction of brain tissue. This ultimately will likely result in enormous levels of AIDS virus-induced dementia.

4. *National health care system in shambles.* The rapidly increasing influx of dying AIDS patients, many suffering with progressive dementia, portends disastrous repercussions for medical care centers. "I can already see the whole hospital system falling apart at the edges", says Dr. Martin Lange of St. Luke's Roosevelt Hospital in New York City.[6]

As of 1982, there were 6,915 hospitals in the United States. 5863 or 85 percent of these are short-term facilities, generally involving patients with stays of thirty days or less. The first ten thousand patients with AIDS will have spent 1,667,900 days in the hospital prior to death.[7] This averages out to a hospital stay totalling 167 days per AIDS patient. Seventy-five percent of all AIDS patients have been seen by only 280 of the acute care hospitals in the United States.[8] Many of these facilities will soon be overwhelmed by the rising influx of new AIDS patients.

Nationally, the number of hospital beds available totaled 1,360,000. On the average, 76 percent of these beds are occupied nationwide. In New York, 88 percent of the beds were occupied on the average in 1982.[9] This leaves 326,000 beds left unoccupied nationwide at any given point during the year.

It should be kept in mind that many of these hospitals are not equipped to handle on a long-term basis the heavy demands on staff and resources required by AIDS patients. Many AIDS patients grow progressively unable to take care of themselves as their condition worsens. Given the forthcoming prospect of another four to five hundred thousand terminally ill AIDS patients, 40 percent or more of whom are likely to be brain-impaired, it is not difficult to perceive why hospital officials see the whole hospital system collapsing under the load. In April of 1986, members of the Health and Public Policy Committee, American College of Physicians, and the Infectious Diseases Society of America stated:

> The neurologic and encephalopathic manifestations of AIDS are being recognized increasingly, and they raise the specter of chronic neurologic disability, possibly requiring institutional care for an unknown number of patients.[10]

With the continuing exponential growth of AIDS infection threatening to raise casualties into the millions, the implosion of the national health care system seems inevitable. Specialized facilities to handle the rapidly increasing influx of dying patients will have to be arranged as existing medical centers become overcrowded.

At present, AIDS patients in some hospitals are being placed in the same rooms or wards with immunocompromised non-AIDS patients (cancer and/or transplant patients etc.) without the latter being informed. This is an unethical and dangerous violation of the protocol called for in treating AIDS patients. The Council on Scientific affairs of the American Medical Association has stated: "The ... patient with AIDS ... should not be in contact with other immunocompromised persons."[11]

5. *Devastation of the Social Security system.* Ninety percent of all AIDS patients thus far have been between the ages of twenty and forty-nine. Four to five hundred thousand persons in this age bracket dying over the next several years will cripple the tax base of workers necessary to provide for present and future recipients of Social Security. In addition, as soon as a person is diagnosed with AIDS he or she immediately becomes eligible for receiving Social Security disability income. In many cases, private insurance coverage is lost due to unemployment. AIDS patients can then become eligible for Medicare or Medicaid. With the direct medical outlay per patient averaging $147,000, resource funds will rapidly become exhausted. Instead of having millions of young and middle-aged workers providing needed revenue for it, the system's resources will be drained by an expanding population of young and middle-aged dependents.

6. *Social and economic chaos.* The repercussions on society of millions of Americans dying of AIDS over the next decade is difficult to fathom. The suffering of the dying combined with the grief of the survivors is an almost incomprehensible portrait of human misery. Although paling in comparison to the staggering toll in human life, the economic consequences will be shattering. A recent report illustrates the staggering economic impact that the AIDS epidemic has begun to have.

Acquired immunodeficiency syndrome (AIDS) is a serious, fatal disease affecting a relatively young population and has a great economic impact. Expenditures for hospitalization and economic losses from disability and premature death were estimated for the first 10,000 patients with AIDS reported in the United States. Extrapolation of data from surveys done in New York City, Philadelphia, and San Francisco suggests that these 10,000 patients with AIDS will require an estimated 1.6 million days in the hospital, resulting in over $1.4 billion in expenditures. Losses incurred for the 8,387 years of work that will be lost from disability and from the premature death of the 10,000 patients will be over $4.8 billion. The total economic burden of the AIDS epidemic will continue to rise as the number of diagnosed cases increases.[12]

Both private and public industry will be devastated by the loss of millions of qualified personnel. The loss of hundreds of billions of dollars of private capital and federal income tax revenue will wreak havoc on the national economy.

Millions upon millions of our nation's men, women and children dying in agony while slowly going mad; our national health care system in shambles; our Social Security programs utterly depleted; the economic and social lifeblood of our nation drained away as the population is decimated: this is the looming specter which will become stark reality if the AIDS epidemic progresses unchecked. Dr. Slaff comments:

> The AIDS virus shows every sign of being just as deadly as the plague during the Middle Ages. We are on a crash course with reality. This is not a practice run. There is no second chance. AIDS may be to the twentieth century what the Black Plague was to the fourteenth century.

The alarm must be sounded, loudly and persuasively. If it is not, the conclusion is inescapable: millions may die.[13]

CHAPTER SEVEN

THE MAJOR OBSTACLE TO HALTING AIDS SPREAD: "ACQUIRED INTEGRITY DEFICIENCY SYNDROME"

Plagues are not new. They have been encountered in every age and among every nationality: syphilis among the Spanish, bubonic plague among the French, tuberculosis among the Eskimos, polio in America.

What is new are efforts by medically unsophisticated politicians and attorneys to dictate policy in regard to an illness that has the potential for wreaking a devastation such as has not been seen encountered on this planet for hundreds of years.[1]
—Dr. Richard Restak, *Washington Post.*

The AIDS epidemic is being treated in a markedly different manner from other great plagues of the past. Other far less virulent venereal diseases have been met with greater efforts at control and prevention than has AIDS.

How Other Devastating Plagues Have Been Handled in the Past

There has been a consistent philosophy underlying measures taken to halt other deadly contagious epidemics in the past: namely, every reasonable effort must be taken to prevent those already infected from transmit-

141

ting the disease at risk to others. In brief, other plagues have been handled as follows:

Bubonic plague: rats carrying infected ticks were exterminated. Infected humans were isolated from those still healthy.

Yellow fever: isolation of those infected; eradication of mosquito breeding grounds.

Smallpox: isolation of those infected from those still healthy.

Dr. Restak explains:

> Throughout history true humanitarianism has traditionally involved the compassionate but firm segregation of those afflicted with communicable diseases from those who are well. By carrying out such a policy, diseases have been contained.[2]

Control of "Classic" Venereal Disease: Many younger Americans may not recall that a few decades ago, prior to the discovery of antibiotics, syphilis was incurable and often resulted after many years in the gradual but progressive destruction of the central nervous system, dementia (insanity), heart disease, crippling joint disease, blindness and death.

> There is a sexually transmitted disease with a very long incubation period, that is life threatening, and incurable. AIDS? No, syphilis prior to 1945. It was defeated by routine epidemiologic techniques. Everyone was tested when hospitalized, married, or inducted into the armed forces until the affected were identified, counseled, and all contacts followed.[3]

Left untreated for a prolonged length of time, syphilis and gonorrhea still have serious medical consequences for those infected. Most women who contract gonorrhea frequently have no symptoms or symptoms so mild that the disease goes unnoticed. Untreated gonorrhea is a major cause of pelvic inflammatory disease (PID) and ectopic pregnancy. PID can require surgical treatment sometimes up to and including a hysterectomy. PID causes 100,000 women to become sterile annually and currently involves hospitalization of about 300,000 women per year.[4] The medical consequence of untreated gonorrhea among women is one of the reasons health officials attempt contact tracing of persons diagnosed with the disease.

Although highly treatable and far less devastating than AIDS, diagnosed cases of syphilis and gonorrhea are still reported to the CDC. Physicians report the cases to appropriate local public health authorities as soon as the diseases are diagnosed so contact tracing can be done. They do not wait until a person has reached the end stages of gonorrhea or tertiary syphilis in order to report the disease.

How AIDS Has Been Handled

1. The CDC only requires reporting of persons who have developed "full-blown", end-stage AIDS. The present CDC definition of AIDS does not include AIDS virus-induced dementia apart from severe immune suppression. AIDS virus-induced tuberculosis is not included. Cases of pre-AIDS are not reported. Persons diagnosed as being asymptomatically infected and capable of transmitting the disease to others are not reported.
2. Most local health authorities do not employ contact tracing for those diagnosed in any stage of AIDS.
3. Efforts to close down the prime breeding grounds of

AIDS contagion (homosexual bathhouses and clubs) have with a few exceptions been almost nonexistent. Any attempts made have occurred very late in the course of the epidemic and have been strongly opposed even by some health officials.

4. Steps which should have been taken to protect the blood supply from contamination with hepatitis B could have largely prevented cases of transfusion-related AIDS. No action was taken to prevent contamination with AIDS until widespread transmission of AIDS infection among users of large quantities of blood products and others had already occurred.

5. National health officials have not informed the public of the crucial fact that AIDS is a lentivirus.

There is a wall of highly-politicized inertia preventing the true facts regarding the nature of AIDS from being made known and impeding practical measures from being taken to stave off its spread. This lethal barrier stems from the inability of major health and political officials and others to reconcile their philosophical presuppositions regarding the nature of human sexuality with the empirical contradiction of the epidemiology of AIDS and other virulent diseases.

AIDS Control and the Medical Establishment

Dr. Selma Dritz of the San Francisco Department of Health, in a 1980 editorial addressing the medical aspects of homosexuality, was, unbeknownst at the time, delineating the conditions and attitudes fostering the brewing AIDS epidemic as well:

With the relaxation of traditional moral restraints and the emergence of more permissive modes of social and sexual interplay in the past ten years, some major cities have acquired large, highly visible homosexual communities. This concentration has produced more opportunities for frequent sexual contacts between homosexual men. In a recent profile of one sample of homosexual patients with sexually transmitted diseases, investigators reported that these men visited public bath houses an average of several times per week and had an average of two to three sexual contacts per visit, largely with anonymous partners. . . .

An average of 10 *percent of all patients and asymptomatic contacts reported to the San Francisco Department of Health because of positive fecal samples or cultures for ameba, giardia, and shigella infections were employed as food handlers in public establishments;* almost 5 per cent of those whom we could reach confirmed that an estimated 60 to 70 per cent of these food handlers were homosexual men. Sources of their infections were either food or sexual contact between male roommates, or oral or anal intercourse between partners who had no food contact. Hepatitis B, a parenteral rather than enteric infection, is considered by some investigators to be transmitted by "parenteral injection" of saliva or semen positive for B antigen through breaks in anal or rectal mucosa during anilingual contact ["scat"] or proctogenital intercourse [sodomy].

Infections in the homosexual community that are not transmitted sexually may also on occasion present a potential problem for the wider population of a city. An outbreak of airborne scarlet fever occurred among homosexual men in San Francisco in 1976 and was identified by the Centers for Disease Control as due to the very rare beta-hemolytic steptococcus A, combination T-Type 6/23. Some adolescent boys attending a local junior high school were known to be active in the homosexual community, and the potential sweep of a previously foreign strain of streptococcus through the large student body posed an immediate threat. Whether the failure of the outbreak to materialize was due even in part to quick action by public health and school officials, or to sheer luck, is one of those questions that epidemiologists often wish they could answer. . . .

Solution of the problem of sexually transmitted disease will require more than effective treatment of active disease in individual patients, because there are many asymptomatic carriers of pathogenic organisms in all sectors of the population. We need effective education for both physicians and the public about the "new" sexually transmitted diseases. We need more rapid and reliable laboratory techniques for diagnosis. We need more effective medication to treat the diseases and to eradicate the asymptomatic carrier states. *We need vaccines that will create sufficient widespread immunity against endemic infections to interrupt transmission of the pathogens by all routes*[5] [emphasis added].

Dr. John C. Fletcher, Assistant for Bioethics at the National Institutes of Health, in a March 1985 editorial applauding the decision of a physician to perform artificial insemination in a lesbian, underscores the ethical world view held by many in the national health establishment:

The weight of traditional religious ethics . . . is clearly against the physician's choice because of the view that the oneness of God is the foundation for the exclusive marriage union of only males and females and the ultimate source of security for the parent child bond. In this view, to act otherwise, as in performing artificial insemination itself or permitting lesbian parenthood, is to disorder God's creation and promote alienation.

Nevertheless he states:

> I agree that ... there are no independent moral rules governing sex. Alternatives to heterosexuality are not evil in themselves, nor do these choices render one intrinsically incapable of being a responsible parent.[6]

This view of the nature of human sexuality has been the driving impetus behind the palliative pansexual guidelines for preventing AIDS issued by health officials. According to the latest advisories espoused by many public health officials, since no one knows who is asymptomatically carrying the AIDS virus everyone in society, married and single, heterosexuals, bisexuals, homosexuals etc. must begin to practice what are deemed to be "safe sex techniques".[7]

In brief, any activity in which "body fluids or secretions" are exchanged is to be avoided. Condoms are unreliable. Sodomy, fellatio, fisting etc., are now considered "high-risk" activities. Since, in their view, no one can really be expected to remain celibate before marriage or faithful afterward, normal heterosexual intercourse, even with one's own spouse, is to be considered dangerous and should be shunned. Passionate kissing is also risky and must become passé. Everyone must start to adopt dry, sterile techniques for petting and massage if the AIDS epidemic is to be contained.

There is, however, a major practical dilemma in this line of advice. Firstly, the adoption of "safe" techniques are of unproven efficacy in preventing AIDS transmission. With the AIDS virus being exuded from almost every bodily orifice, pore and secretion, probably including sweat, prolonged intimate sexual contact of any kind is potentially lethal.

If the CDC recommendations on avoiding contact

with AIDS-tainted secretions are taken seriously, the only "safe" sex with an AIDS carrier would necessitate wearing surgical gowns and mask, rubber gloves and eye goggles. According to Dr. Luc Montagnier, the genetic variability of the AIDS virus can result in change in modes of transmission. This hardly leaves grounds for glib advice about alleged means of "safe" intimate sexual interaction. Also disturbing is the apparent contradiction to "safe-sex guidelines" issued by the Council on Scientific Affairs of the American Medical Association:

> Sexual contact should be avoided with persons known to have or suspected of having AIDS.[8]

Secondly, even if these allegedly "safe" guidelines were theoretically efficacious and adhered to by everyone in society, where does that leave heterosexual procreation of the human race? Relegated to the Brave New World of rows of artificially inseminated test tube babies raised in hermetically sealed laboratories? Apart from its questionable ethical aspects, attempts to produce an infant in vitro have proven abysmally short-lived. Strictly followed, universal adoption of practices excluding the act of procreation would result in the self-extinction of mankind.

In addition to this type of blatant inanity, there has been an alarming trend in the medical establishment to violate safe guidelines in protecting patients and medical personnel from AIDS contagion. The official testimony of Candice Comstive, R.N., before the Houston City Council, September 25, 1985, illustrates how widespread these unethical and dangerous violations of protocol have become:

My name is Candice Comstive. I was educated at Houston Community College and graduated from the University of Texas School of Nursing (Houston) in March, 1982, with a Bachelor's Degree in Nursing.

I was employed at Memorial City Medical Center as of November 5, 1984. I was hired to work full time on 2 North, the Oncology (cancer) floor. Nothing was mentioned concerning caring for AIDS patients. I was unaware that this was expected from all nursing personnel.

Since that time, many incidents have occurred which have caused me to resign September 23, 1985. I will highlight several of them below:

(1) I was assigned AIDS patients without being informed of their disease until days later. I have talked with other nurses who have expressed similar complaints.

(2) Isolation does not mean separation. AIDS patients and/or "Suspected AIDS" patients (those having the HTVL-III antibody in their blood but no recurrent infections), are housed among the general hospital population.

While on the same floor as other patients, I have had AIDS victims that have not been placed on any type of isolation technique whatsoever. Others may be placed on a type of isolation titled "blood 7 secretion precautions." This means that gloves are the only protective garb required to be worn *if* personnel feel they will be coming into contact with body secretions (blood, urine, feces, mucus, semen etc.).

(3) AIDS patients are not confined to their rooms. Many walk through the halls and even share the same kitchen that the nursing staff, patients and their families use.

I had one AIDS patient in January 1985 who was placed on *"strict isolation"*. He was in the kitchen at 7:30 A.M. pouring himself coffee which was not unusual. I suggested he return to his room and with that he turned and vomited on me and the kitchen as well. I changed into "scrubs" and returned to my assignment of patients for the day. An unsuspecting "house-cleaning" employee with mop in hand cleaned up the mess left on the cabinets and floor.

(4) Care for AIDS patients as they progress in the disease is quite similar to what one would find in a skilled nursing home. There are frequent episodes of diarrhea and incontinence of urine. The tremendous weakening of their bodies makes it almost impossible for them to walk. A nurse is responsible for keeping their beds and rooms clean, feeding them, and washing their bodies (plastic gloves that come up to the wrist are provided for the nurse—I have found they break apart and leak easily). Working with needles is also expected as nurses are required to give shots and start intravenous solutions if they are ordered by the physicians. Needle sticks are not uncommon accidents. Contaminated needles have been proven to transfer the AIDS virus.

(5) We have no designated rooms for AIDS patients throughout the hospital. A room will be used for an AIDS patient. He will then be discharged, transferred or die. That evening a cancer patient conceivably could be admitted to the same room. *Rooms at the end of the hall used for AIDS patients are also used by pediatric patients.*

(6) All departments from housekeeping to volunteers, lab technicians to physical therapists are involved in caring for AIDS patients. No one to my knowledge has been given a choice nor has anyone been screened on a regular basis for the AIDS virus.

(7) My mother and I voiced our fears and grievances to administration September 20, 1985. It was suggested that I look for work elsewhere due to my expressed concerns. Administration added they did not think I would be able to find work in any hospital though because AIDS is being treated in the same manner all

over. Nurses employed elsewhere have verbally vali-
dated that statement.

(8) All health care personnel are faced with the same
ultimatum—If you do not want to care for AIDS patients
do not seek employment at a hospital. After being educated and trained over a four-year period, I am being
made to seek employment outside the hospital as the
only alternative to my choices and desires. Legally there
is nothing I can do but resign[9] (emphasis added).

Similar accounts are being reported from all over the
United States. Yale University's Dr. Lowell Levin, commenting on studies indicating that some two million
patients contract dangerous infections (not necessarily
AIDS) each year while being treated in American hospitals states: "It sounds like a joke, but a hospital is no
place for a sick person to be."[10]

Judicial and Political Activism and the Rise of AIDS

In many instances, rulings at various levels of the nation's
judicial and political system have helped foster conditions abetting the growth and rapid spread of the AIDS
epidemic.

In its 1981 decision holding the state's antisodomy
law to be unconstitutional, the highest court of the
State of New York concluded that there was no rational
basis for the law and then said:

Nor is any such basis as supplied by the claims advanced
by the prosecution—that a prohibition against consensual sodomy will prevent physical harm which might
otherwise befall the participants, will uphold public morality and will protect the institution of marriage. Com-

mendable though these objectives clearly are, there is nothing on which to base a conclusion that they are achieved by section 130.38 [prohibition of consensual sodomy] of the Penal Law. *No showing has been made, even in references tendered in the briefs, that physical injury is a common or even occasional consequence of the prohibited conduct . . .* [emphasis added].[11]

Interestingly, an editorial in the renowned *New England Journal of Medicine* published one year prior to the ruling had stated:

Oral and anal intercourse present physicians with surgical as well as medical problems, ranging from anal fissures and impaction of foreign bodies in the rectum to major diagnostic dilemmas. Infection in traumatized rectal mucosa and in amebic or herpetic ulcers above the level of the anal ring may produce formations that mimic rectal carcinoma.[12]

It is ironic that in 1981, at the same time as the court was declaring sodomy to be an innocuous practice, the AIDS epidemic was picking up steam in New York City's bathhouses as a direct consequence of homosexual men anonymously sodomizing one another at breakneck levels of promiscuity.

New York City now has the dubious distinction of being the AIDS capital of the Western world. Having the state's antisodomy law previously declared unconstitutional has stymied efforts to close down establishments which foster the proliferation of AIDS by encouraging mass anonymous homosexual promiscuity.

After years of laissez-faire policy permitting the AIDS epidemic to spread unimpeded, the New York State Public Health Council finally decided to pass a resolution calling for the closing of establishments permitting "high-risk" homosexual activity (sodomy and fellatio) on their premises. Although a few of the more notorious clubs have for the nonce been closed, others remain open. The homosexual activists and civil libertarians are now raising the hue and cry that the prohibition of these activities has been declared unconstitutional and they are seeking to have them reopened.[13] Similar objections have been raised in other states which have had their antisodomy statutes overturned by the courts.

In Minneapolis, the City Council passed sweeping legislation banning any private employer, including religious institutions or churches, from any type of selectivity in hiring based on individual same-sex preference. In response to complaints to the city's Civil Rights Commission, the Big Brothers organization, which provides older males as role models for fatherless boys, were compelled to actively solicit homosexuals as volunteers. They were also forbidden to mention the applicant's same-sex preference to the child's parent. Membership in the paedophile North American Man/Boy Love Association (NAMBLA) is not considered an inherent bar to becoming a Big Brother to little boys.

A well-known evangelical Bible college in the city reportedly has refrained from expelling known practicing homosexual students for fear of being brought up on charges before the Council.

The Minneapolis Ordinance has been hailed by homosexual activists and civil libertarians as an outstanding prototype for similar types of legislation being initiated at the state and federal levels.

In light of the host of virulent communicable diseases endemic in the homosexual community, one particular section from the ordinance is especially noteworthy:

> It is determined that discriminatory practices based on . . . sex *or affectional or sexual preference* with respect to employment, labor union membership, housing accommodations, property rights, education, public accommodations, and public services, or any of them, tend to create and intensify conditions of . . . ill health, . . . lawlessness, and vice and adversely affect the public health, safety, order, convenience and general welfare . . . [14] [emphasis theirs].

Paradoxically, this legislation resulted in the prosecution of the owner of a family health club chain for ejecting patrons found soliciting and engaging in "high-risk" homosexual acts on the premises of his Minneapolis club.

Arthur Owens, the club owner, explained the need for regulations restricting homosexual behavior. "We caught homosexuals committing sex acts. Our customers complained that they were being propositioned." Eventually he was fined and forced to close the club for refusing to permit these activities to continue.[15]

As the courts and state and local legislatures extirpated traditional mores from the law, they paved the legislative way for conditions abetting the spread of AIDS and other venereal diseases.

Charles Rice, professor of constitutional law at the University of Notre Dame Law School, incisively comments:

> The positive law and judicial decisions reflect the prevailing morality, but they also perform an educative role in shaping the moral views of the community. . . .
>
> The AIDS epidemic shows the wisdom of the common law position which was derived from the religious condemnation of homosexuality. The common law for four and one-half centuries affirmed that the legitimization of homosexual activity is contrary to the public good.[16]

Media Censorship and the AIDS Epidemic

The major media have been consistent in their censorship of vital information regarding the AIDS epidemic. The nature of the AIDS agent—i.e., its being a lentivirus, and all that implies in terms of mortality and routes of transmission—has been virtually blacked out. The crucial long-established fact that infection with the AIDS virus itself is deadly has been repeatedly downplayed and outrightly contradicted. Major studies giving evidence of the potential of casual transmission have gone completely unreported, while toxic "cures" and groundless optimism regarding vaccine development have made front-page news. Every effort is being made to divert attention from the major risk group involved in conveying the epidemic.

On January 22, 1986 the Associated Press reported:

> The subject of AIDS ... is now becoming a hot topic in entertainment programming. In the next two weeks, TV characters will contract AIDS on the medical show "Saint Elsewhere", the youth-oriented sitcom "Mr. Belvedere" and the light drama series, "Hotel". Most AIDS cases have occurred in male homosexuals and intravenous drug abusers, but the three series chose to create stories around examples of AIDS transmissions that are statistically much smaller [e.g., Dr. Bobby Caldwell will get AIDS from a female carrier of the disease after they've had sexual relations].[17]

One national magazine commented:

> AIDS has created a new journalistic genre: the sufferings of the AIDS victim. A young man is introduced, who has twelve, six, three months to live. There are descriptions of his symptoms, his mood (variable), and

his prospects (nil). Spliced into the account are tributes
to his talents and to his human qualities, so soon to be
extinguished. There may be some discussion of the larger
issue involved (invariably as they are framed by the
homosexual establishment: Why haven't doctors or the
government done more? Who is to blame?). But the
focus is on the individual sufferer.

Such stories are affecting, for the subject of an untimely
and wasting death must excite sympathy. One thing,
though, is typically left out — the culture of homosexual
promiscuity in which the disease has flourished in this
country. One account, in *New York* magazine, touched
the subject almost unconsciously. The irony of the victim's
plight, it was made clear, was that his sexual life had
been particularly stable. He had had one lover for ten
years; he had sown his wild oats. Except that, once a
week, the two would spend the night apart.

Once every week is half a hundred partners — *lovers*
seems hardly the word — a year. Ten years of that takes
you halfway to Don Giovanni's *mil e tre* [1003]. In a
heterosexual, that is promiscuous. And that is nothing
compared to the tempo of the parks, the subway toilets,
the bathhouses, where casual couplers might run through
a dozen or more partners a day — the rate of prostitutes.[18]

A recent report published in *Public Opinion,* a magazine of the American Institute for Public Policy Research
in Washington, D.C., describes the ethical views regarding the nature of sexuality held by leaders in the media
establishment. The report was written by the research
team of Robert Lichter (political scientist at George
Washington University), Stanley Rothman (professor at
Smith College) and Linda Lichter (research associate at
George Washington University). The findings are the
result of extensive interviews with 104 of the nation's
leading television broadcasters. The eclectic survey

included only persons who were associated with two or more successful prime-time series, including "some of the most experienced and respected members of the craft. Many have been honored with Emmy awards, and a few are household names."

Eighty percent of those interviewed do not regard homosexual relations as wrong. Eighty-six percent support the rights of homosexuals to teach in the public schools. Fifty-one percent do not regard adultery as wrong.

The survey also revealed that those interviewed "seek to move their audience toward their vision of the good society".[19]

The Role of the Homosexual Movement in the AIDS Disinformation Campaign

HOMOSEXUAL ACTIVISM AND THE MEDICAL ESTABLISHMENT

On September 23, 1983, a medical task force at the University of California, San Francisco, developed infection control guidelines for patients with AIDS. Their guidelines, presented in the *New England Journal of Medicine,* were developed to address two main concerns: the potential transmissibility of a putative AIDS agent (HTLV–III was not yet defined as the agent) and the transmissibility of opportunistic pathogens (agents for AIDS-related infections). The guidelines stated in part:

> Transmission of the disease appears to have an epidemiologic pattern similar to hepatitis B. . . . This suggests that the disease may be transmitted by blood, tissue,

and secretions or excretions that may contain blood (or the virus). . . .

Pregnant employees should not engage in the direct care of patients with AIDS, because of the potential for birth defects from cytomegalovirus and the potentially large amounts of this virus that may be disseminated from such patients. . . .

Cardiopulmonary Resuscitation in the Hospital Setting

Resuscitation bags, or disposable devices for mouth-to-mouth cardiopulmonary resuscitation (CPR) should be available for every patient and should be kept at the bedside of patients with AIDS and other patients with potentially transmissible infections—for example, hepatitis B infection or tuberculosis. When such a CPR device is available, the employee is obliged to administer CPR. The decision to withhold direct mouth-to-mouth resuscitation from a patient with AIDS when a CPR device is not available is solely that of the individual employee.

CPR training should include instruction in the use of disposable devices to prevent mouth-to-mouth contact between the resuscitator and the patient. Hospital employees with documented AIDS should be excused from participating in the two-person manikin phase of the CPR training program. Consideration should be given to revising the recertification procedures to eliminate mouth-to-mouth contact with manikins during the two-person training phase for all persons undergoing CPR recertification. Employees with AIDS should not, however, be excused from other phases of the training program, nor should they be discouraged from becoming recertified in CPR.

. . . Although there are good epidemiologic data to support the occurrence of a transmissible agent of AIDS in blood, there is no current evidence for its presence in saliva. In performing cardiopulmonary resuscitation the resuscitator may come into contact with saliva containing blood or vomitus or both. This exposure to blood may serve as a way of transmitting the AIDS agent. For these reasons, the task force members *felt strongly* that these issues should be addressed in the guidelines.[20]

A few months later, the *New England Journal of Medicine* presented a letter responding to the above guidelines.

To the Editor: As a representative of BI POL (a bisexual/lesbian/gay political-action organization in San Francisco), I want to express the deep disturbance of the bisexual community regarding your recent article on infection control guidelines for hospital personnel working with persons with the acquired immunodeficiency syndrome (AIDS). . . .

What were alarming . . . were the guidelines for cardio-pulmonary resuscitation, which could be taken for an employee's refusal to carry out an emergency life-saving procedure on the basis of the health worker's fear of contracting AIDS. . . . What can be the justification for making an exception in the case of persons with AIDS?

These guidelines allow employee's irrational or vague fears to determine their obligation to take action in an emergency, instead of recognizing the hospital's responsibility for ensuring that all its patients receive appropriate care. . . . [21]

The above letter was referred to the authors of the AIDS infection preventive guidelines that were questioned. The doctors responded in the same issue:

To the Editor: The infection-control guidelines developed by the University of California, San Francisco, Task Force on AIDS represented a working document. We presented a consensus of opinions expressed by many people with divergent backgrounds and perspectives. The guidelines were formulated to assist health-care workers in the hospital setting in the care of patients with AIDS. After further deliberation the Task Force agreed that the statement regarding mouth-to-mouth resuscitation—i.e., that decision to provide mouth-to-mouth resuscitation is a personal one—was unnecessary. Therefore, it has been deleted from the final report submitted by the Task Force to the office of the dean. . . . [22]

If the members of the Task Force had not been quite so hasty in capitulating to the objections of the homosexual activists, they would have soon found additional medical support for their initial "strongly felt" caution on performing mouth-to-mouth CPR. On October 26, 1984, researchers reported in *Nature* that they had isolated HTLV–III from the saliva of four ARC patients and two healthy homosexual males.

> HTLV–III . . . is efficiently transmitted by cell-free virus. . . . Cells producing virus, as well as cell-free virus, were observed in the saliva of the patients described here. . . . The recovery of HTLV–III from saliva suggests that direct contact with this body fluid should be avoided since saliva . . . could facilitate horizontal transmission.[23]

Also, the Task Force stated that "pregnant employees should not engage in the direct care of patients with AIDS. . . . " Where did that leave the pregnant patient being treated by a hospital employee with AIDS? Conspicuously absent in the initial "safe" AIDS infection control guidelines is the mention of the risk of hospital employees with AIDS performing mouth-to-mouth resuscitation on non-AIDS patients (e.g., pregnant patients, immunosuppressed cancer or transplant patients etc.). They state: "Employees with AIDS . . . should not . . . be discouraged from becoming recertified in CPR." In retrospect, now that it is known that

AIDS virus is contained in saliva and that severe lung diseases (including tuberculosis and chronic lymphoid interstitial pneumonitis [CLIP]) can be complications of AIDS infection, the implied sanction of health care workers with AIDS giving mouth-to-mouth resuscitation to patients appears rash and precipitous at best.

In addition to the type of influence exerted by homosexual activist groups in shaping "safe" AIDS infection control guidelines, it appears that these groups have played a major role in formulating public health policy regarding AIDS on the national level. The National Coalition of Gay STD [sexually transmitted disease] Services was established in 1979 in Chicago "by representatives from several of the nation's gay STD services and interested individuals: Chicago's Howard Brown Memorial Clinic, Milwaukee's Gay Peoples Union Venereal Disease Clinic, New York's Gay Men's Health Project and St. Mark's Clinic, Washington, D.C.'s Whitman-Walker Gay Men's Venereal Disease Clinic, and gay representatives (unaffiliated) from Denver and New Orleans".[24]

This organization has established a very close working relationship with the Centers for Disease Control (CDC), a U.S. government agency.[25]

This relationship is very beneficial to the homosexual movement in terms of recognition and funding. The coalition itself has reported that it serves as the vehicle through which the CDC receives information for the preparation of its VD research agenda. The control of this information is crucial in the allocation of public research funds. As happens in so many other areas of public funding, the recipients of the funds come to exercise a key role in the allocation of the funding. In

this case, it is homosexual organizations that are involved
in these activities.[26]

HOMOSEXUAL ACTIVISM AND THE MEDIA

According to the January–February 1981 issue of *It's
Time* (newsletter of the National Gay Task Force
[NGTF]): "Work is progressing with NGTF's plans to
target major American institutions for educational
campaigns designed to make a positive impact on their
perceptions of lesbians and gay men. Dr. Charles Hitchcock, the NGTF Public Education Consultant, reports
that he has made religious, media and educational institutions the foci of the program." In a subsequent issue
of *It's Time,* Hitchcock elaborated on the ways in
which the NGTF expected to effect this social change.
He added:

> Individual programs are being designed for each spe-
> cific institution. Components include a history of each
> institution's attitudes or policies on gay rights, identifica-
> tion of institutional decision-makers and decision making
> processes, and a curriculum for an educational (training)
> program with appropriate materials and resource people
> identified. *A prime example would be that of a national
> television network* where, because of the lack of any
> stated policy or educational materials concerned with
> gay issues, individuals are left to their own personal
> whim or prejudice in dealing with gay stories and news
> items. In targeting such an institution for our program,
> *we would,* through staff meetings, educational seminars
> and the development of relevant educational materials,
> *hope to have a major positive impact on how that institu-
> tion deals with gay concerns—both internally and in its
> entertainment programs and news coverage*[27] [emphasis
> added].

Heterophobia and Sex Education
in the Public Schools

One of the stated major goals of the homosexual movement is to have homosexuality taught in the public schools as a healthy alternative sexual lifestyle. In the view of proponents of this movement, for young people (or anyone else) to be exclusively fixated on heterosexual relations is perceived as a threat to establishing a pansexual society. Any suggestion that a monogamous heterosexual relationship is the ideal model for sexual expression is regarded with trepidation and contempt. Heterophobia, the fear of heterosexuality or expressing an exclusive preference for opposite-sex relations in one's self or others, has become a pervasive element in many of the nation's public school sex education classes. In New York City for example, the Board of Education has published a new Sex Education Program (SEP) that is 293 pages long. One prominent attorney and children's rights activist comments:

> That's about 283 pages longer than is necessary to instruct pupils in the facts of life; the rest is classroom fun and games designed to subject pupils to psychological treatment, to require pupils to reveal information about sex behavior and attitudes, to require pupils to discuss psychological problems potentially embarassing to the student and his family's privacy, and to elicit critical appraisals of other individuals with whom the pupils have close relationships. . . .
>
> . . . being a public school course, SEP does not tell pupils that premarital sex is wrong; the teacher would be forbidden to do that. Instead, the pupil is instructed "to identify and evaluate the choices involved in sexual expression". The choices then listed for the student are

"abstinence, sexual fantasy, masturbation, hugging, kissing, petting, exploration, intercourse, nocturnal emis-
sion or wet dreams, sexual preference, homosexual
preference, homosexual experience, gay, lesbian, bisexual,
transvestite, transsexual" (p. 137).

SEP forces explicit discussions of sexuality and genitalia on little children at the kindergarten and primary
grade levels (p. 30).

A persistent undercurrent of SEP is its attempt to
teach pupils to be tolerant of homosexuals. "Experimental
sex play" with persons of the same sex is described as
"not unusual" among 5th and 6th grade children (p. 63).
"Homosexual experimentation" is described as a normal
behavior of 14-16 year olds (p. 19).[28]

This type of teaching is consistent with the goals
of groups like the North American Man/Boy Love
Association. NAMBLA is an organization dedicated to
the legalization of paedophilia or sex with children—in
their case, young boys in particular.

Legislative Goals of the Homosexual Movement

In 1972, the National Coalition of Gay Organizations
adopted what was called the "1972 Gay Rights Platform".
This platform has been the manifesto undergirding
homosexual political activism. Some of the stated goals
are highly pertinent in light of the AIDS epidemic.

DEMANDS

Federal:

1. Amend all federal Civil Rights Acts, other legislation
    and government controls to prohibit discrimination in

employment, housing, public accommodations and public services. . . .

6. Federal encouragement and support for sex education courses, prepared and taught by gay women and men, presenting homosexuality as a valid, healthy preference and lifestyle as a viable alternative to heterosexuality.

State:

2. Repeal of all state laws prohibiting private sexual acts involving consenting persons. . . .

3. Repeal all state laws prohibiting solicitation for private voluntary sexual liaisons; and laws prohibiting prostitution, both male and female.

4. Enactment of legislation prohibiting insurance companies and any other state-regulated enterprises from discriminating because of sexual orientation. . . .

5. Enactment of legislation so that child custody, adoption, visitation rights, foster parenting, and the like shall not be denied because of sexual orientation. . . .

7. Repeal of all laws governing the age of consent.[29]

Summed up, the ongoing tenaciously held goal of the homosexual movement is:

Acceptance of homosexual acts as a normal variant of human behavior and of homosexuality as an alternative lifestyle.[30]

In New York and San Francisco, 70 to 90 percent of practicing male homosexuals are estimated to be infected with and infectious for the AIDS virus.[31] On June 7, 1985, the CDC issued recommendations for the prevention of hepatitis B. One particular section is especially enlightening:

Homosexually active men. Susceptible homosexually active men should be vaccinated regardless of their ages

or duration of their homosexual practices. It is important to vaccinate persons as soon as possible after their
homosexual activity begins.[32]

The implications of the CDC advice are chillingly
clear. All persons who have been or will be involved
in male homosexual behavior are susceptible to become
infected with hepatitis B and should be vaccinated.
The prevalence and routes of AIDS transmission parallel
those of hepatitis B, especially in regards to male homosexual behavior. There is no vaccine to ward off AIDS
infection. Any boy or man, therefore, entering the homosexual subculture can expect to become infected with
AIDS. Given what is presently known about the dire
long-term consequences of AIDS infection, entrance
into the homosexual subculture spells devastating medical consequences and a probable death sentence.

Dr. William Haseltine, a leading AIDS researcher
at the Harvard Medical School in Boston, ominously
asserts, "We must be prepared to anticipate that the
vast majority of those now infected will ultimately, over
a period of five to ten years, develop life-threatening
illness."[33]*

The pathological consequences of homosexual acts

---

*For a more detailed discussion of the grave implications of
AIDS virus infection in high-risk group members, the reader is
referred to the study in the April 1986 *Annals of Internal Medicine,*
by Dr. Robert Gallo and other researchers, "Long-Term Seropositivity
for Human T-Lymphotropic Virus Type III in Homosexual Men
without the Acquired Immunodeficiency Syndrome: Development
of Immunologic and Clinical Abnormalities" (pp. 496–500). The
medium and long-range prognosis, based on the most current
evidence, appears quite grim. The researchers conclude: "A high
proportion of persons infected with HTLV-III will develop measur-
able immunologic and clinical abnormalities."

per se, the host of virulent diseases running rife and the pandemic of AIDS in their midst are galling empirical contradictions to the positive image the homosexual movement has been striving to convey. Desperate to prevent this image from being shattered, every effort has been made to impede the truth regarding AIDS being made widely known.

CHAPTER EIGHT

STOPPING THE AIDS JUGGERNAUT

... humanly speaking, had decisive measures been adopted while the disorder existed only in one street, and in a few houses in that street, there can be little doubt, that it might have been very soon extinguished.
— J. H. Powell, *Bring out Your Dead, The Great Plague of Yellow Fever in Philadelphia in* 1793.[1]

Understandably enough, the areas of the United States in which AIDS has grown most rapidly are also those in which local public health officials and politicos are most susceptible to pressure by partisan interest groups at primary risk of conveying the disease.

In Wisconsin, James Pawlisch, a member of the Dane County Board of Health, was dismissed following his comment at a board meeting that homosexual behavior was unnatural and immoral and homosexuals should realize that AIDS is a risk of such behavior.

The Fourth District Court of Appeals upheld his dismissal, noting that Pawlisch's remarks were contrary to the nondiscrimination policy of the county's executive administrator Jonathan Barry and that "commonality of political beliefs with the prevailing policy maker ... is required for the effective performance of an office ... we conclude that speech restrictions do apply."[2]

Dr. Gordon Muir comments:

... even some health officials with serious responsibility for the control of AIDS are acting peculiarly. Such

169

a one is the Dallas County epidemiologist, with whom I discussed the epidemiologically obvious need to close down the Club Dallas Bathhouse. (This establishment, with a reported patronage of over 30,000, has recently been advertising special cheap locker rates for teenagers.) At first he said he was unaware the club was still open, then defended such clubs (it would be "purely political" to close them down).[3]

New York City has generated over a third of all AIDS cases in the United States. In June of 1985, Mayor Edward Koch led the city's annual homosexual liberation parade. Smiling, with arms raised and flashing the victory sign, he was trailed by thousands of homosexual activists, some carrying banners touting the North American Man/Boy Love Association.

The former New York City Commissioner of Public Health, Dr. David Sencer, passionately pleaded with the Surgeon-General not to close homosexual bathhouses but to instead "take a child by the hand and lead him/her to school". The bathhouses "do not spread disease", said Sencer (this despite the national case study indicating homosexual AIDS patients have found 50 percent of their prior sex contacts in bathhouses).[4]

Sencer has also made the AIDS blood screening test illegal for private physicians to use and refused to make any efforts at tracing contacts of infected patients.

"Gays put pressure on the Board of Health to forbid the test", says Dr. Helen Singer Kaplan, head of the Human Sexuality Program at the New York Hospital-Cornell Medical Center. "We would stop the spread of AIDS today if these high-risk people, these Typhoid Marys, would stop spreading the disease. As a physician and scientist, I'm appalled at their wildly having sex and spreading AIDS."[5]

As Dr. Slaff of the National Institutes of Health admits: "There should be some mechanism to prevent and punish this type of behavior."[6]

Federal Action Is Imperative

The prohomosexual political chauvinism which prevails in many municipalities and states has gravely impaired the credibility of local officials in dealing objectively with the AIDS epidemic. High risk carriers of AIDS are being systematically protected and the lives of countless others put in jeopardy by the unwillingness and inability of state and local officials to take effective action to stop its spread.

Federal action is essential if the "Typhoid Mikes and Marys" of the AIDS epidemic are to be prevented from continuing to infect others individually and en masse.

Any suggestion that legal measures should be utilized to combat the AIDS crisis has been met with the objection of ostensible civil libertarians that it is impossible to legislate morality. This contention involves sophistry. All legislation is inextricably interwoven with some underlying system of ethics. Laws against murder and stealing are based on the Mosaic law. Laws against drunk driving are based on the narrow moral view asserting that the right of the general citizenry to live supersedes the "right" of the individual to drive recklessly.

In any civilized society, there must be certain rules of conduct governing human behavior. Although we cherish individual freedom, we have never accepted the notion that it is absolute and without limitation. Despite the libertarian thrust of its opinions, even the Supreme Court of the United States has acknowledged the fact that total freedom would lead to anarchy and the death of freedom. As Justice Oliver Wendell Holmes rightly insisted, no one has the right to shout fire falsely in a crowded theater.[7]

In a sense, it is correct that you cannot legislate an individual's sense of enjoyment in abiding by the law. The potential drunk driver, rapist or thug may never like the fact that his personal preferences are being curtailed by legislative mandate. There will always be those who choose to violate the law and risk the penalties involved.

Nevertheless, legal sanctions do foster a general external obedience, even among those unwillingly inclined. Only an anarchist would contend that because we have individuals who murder, rape, steal and drive while drunk that we should abolish all laws prohibiting such antisocial behavior. If anything, many today would argue that stiffer legislative penalties must be imposed on those who endanger the lives of others.

Likewise, there will always be those who choose to engage in behavior putting themselves and others at risk of AIDS infection. A lack of personal self-preservation and moral responsibility notwithstanding, legal restrictions can significantly curtail the number of opportunities available for these individuals to acquire and disseminate AIDS infection. The so-called "right to privacy" is abrogated when acts done in private result in the spread of a deadly public epidemic. Dr. Restak notes:

> Only sentimentalists refuse to make any distinction between the victims of a scourge and those not presently infected. . . . The threat of AIDS demands from us all a discrimination based on our instinct for survival against a peril, that if not somehow controlled, can

destroy this society. This is a discrimination that recognizes that caution is in order when knowledge is incomplete so that the public interest can be protected....

The humanitarian response to AIDS is exactly the opposite of a humanitarian response to sexism or racism: In the presence of considerable ignorance about the causes and effects of the syndrome, the benefit of the doubt should not be given to the victim of AIDS. This is not a civil rights issue, this is a medical issue. To take a position that the AIDS virus must be eradicated is not to make judgments on morals or lifestyles. It is to say that the AIDS virus has no "civil rights".[8]

Legislative Steps to Halt AIDS Spread

1. *Empower and support the Surgeon General to take practical measures to halt the spread of AIDS.*

Fortunately, there is federal legislation on the books right now which could significantly hinder the unrestricted spread of AIDS contagion by those knowingly spreading the disease. The Federal Code states:

264. *Control of communicable diseases*

(a) The Surgeon General, with the approval of the Administrator [Secretary], is authorized to make and enforce such regulations as in his judgment are necessary to prevent the introduction, transmission, or spread of communicable diseases from foreign countries into the States or possessions, or from one state or possession into any other State or possession....

(d) On recommendation of the National Advisory Health Council, regulations prescribed under this section may provide for the apprehension and examination of any individual reasonably believed to be infected with a communicable disease in a communicable stage and (1) to be moving or about to move from a State to another State; or (2) to be a probable source of infection to individuals who, while infected with such disease in a communicable stage, will be moving from a State to another State. Such regulations may provide that if upon examination any such individual is found to be infected, he may be detained for such time and in such manner as may be reasonabe and necessary. *United States Code Service,* 42 USCS, The Public Health and Welfare.[9]

Infectious tuberculosis is already included under this provision. The signing of an executive order by the President naming the disease at risk is all that is required for the Surgeon General to put the above provisions in effect regarding those who would intentionally put others in danger of acquiring AIDS.

On March 22, 1985, AIDS became subject to the provisions of the Public Health (Control of Disease) Act 1984 in England.

These provisions . . . allow orders to be made for patients who have AIDS to be medically examined and for AIDS patients to be removed to hospital and detained there.[10]

From a public health standpoint this type of exercise of governmental authority is not without warrant:

Most people might agree that government actions designed to protect the health of the public at large are appropriate and proper, even though they may be objectionable to some members of the public. . . . Likewise laws allowing a quarantine in the case of a contagious disease or permitting health authorities to remove a nuisance that poses a danger to public health are generally considered acceptable and desirable public activities. R. Roemer and G. A. McKray, *Legal Aspects of Public Health.* [11]

As a preface to the enacting of further protective legislation, the Surgeon General should be authorized to employ whatever measures are deemed appropriate for restraining the dissemination of AIDS as stated in the Federal Code.

2. *Federal order closing down all known homosexual bathhouses.*

Dr. Frederick P. Siegal in his 1983 book *AIDS: The Medical Mystery* asserts that homosexual bathhouses

> in particular are actively promoting and commercially exploiting anonymous promiscuity, a practice now clearly linked with the transmission of a lethal disease. Anonymous sex is highly risky because unfamiliar sexual partners may be unknowingly or knowingly ill or may have been exposed to others with AIDS, and intercourse with a large number of contacts just multiplies the risks. . . . It could fairly be argued that allowing such hazardous activity to continue betrays official indifference to the lives of gay men, who should be protected by public health services.[12]

In light of research indicating that 65 percent of homosexual men have engaged in heterosexual activity and that 20 percent or more have been or are married, it can be argued that allowing these facilities to remain open also betrays indifference to the lives of the female partners of those attending the bathhouses. Further, some of these bathhouses offer special cheap locker rates to teenagers and younger males encouraging the spread of AIDS among youth.

Passing out condoms, erecting billboards and handing out flyers suggesting that bathhouse patrons "play safely" are missing the point. If you have a dining establishment whose patrons are continually dying of food poisoning, you don't hand out stomach pumps to customers going in—you close the restaurant.

As a first practical step to stemming the most blatant, teeming sources of AIDS contagion, the high-risk homosexual bathhouses and "clubs" must be closed permanently by federal edict.

3. *Federal bans on all high-risk group members from:*
   —*donating blood or plasma.*
   —*contributing semen to sperm banks.*
   —*donating organs.*

The present AIDS blood screening test still permits a certain percentage of those infected with AIDS to slip through the safety net and endanger people's lives. All prospective donors of any of these protected substances must be required to sign a statement under oath that they are not members of a high-risk group. Mandatory high federal penalties would be imposed on violators.

4. *Hospital officials must allow medical personnel to take proper precautions when dealing with AIDS patients. Proper precautions must be taken to protect non-AIDS patients from those with AIDS.*

Some hospital administrations are not permitting personnel to take necessary safety precautions (mask, gown, goggles) in dealing with AIDS patients (so as to avoid "stigmatizing"). Pregnant nurses are not being informed that they are dealing with AIDS patients despite the grave risk to their unborn child. In some hospitals, AIDS patients are being put in the same ward or room with immunocompromised non-AIDS patients. This is a violation of the non-AIDS patient's right to safe care and right to know. Staff and personnel desiring to take precautions for themselves or to inform the non-AIDS patients at risk are threatened with dismissal. These and other practices threatening the lives of noninfected personnel and patients must cease.

5. *Federal registration of all persons diagnosed with full-blown AIDS, pre-AIDS (ARC) and those testing positive with the AIDS blood screening test.*

Contact tracing for prior and present sexual contacts must be implemented.

Persons with serious AIDS virus-induced disease without CDC-defined AIDS or immunosuppression (e.g., AIDS virus-induced dementia and tuberculosis) must be considered included under this definition. Dr. James J. Goedert and other AIDS researchers from the National Cancer Institute and Downstate Medical Center asserted in *Lancet:*

> The strict definition of the acquired immunodeficiency syndrome (AIDS) used by the US Centers for Disease Control for surveillance purposes does not accommodate the wide range of clinical conditions that occur in people infected with human T-lymphotropic virus type III (HTLV-III). . . .
> We propose that infections with *M tuberculosis hominis* in a population at risk of AIDS be included as manifestation of lesser AIDS, at least until sero-epidemiological studies can disprove association with HTLV-III.[13]

Pre-AIDS or ARC patients must be reported. Persons who are shown to be asymptomatically infected must be reported. If any practical efforts are to be made to halt the spread of AIDS infection, it is essential to find out who is infected and take practical steps to prevent these persons from infecting others.

From the standpoint of those who have been unknowingly infected with AIDS, it is essential that they be informed that: 1. they are at risk for developing the disease, and 2. they must take steps to avoid spreading the disease to others.

With a view toward preserving public health, it is absolutely crucial to track down those who may be unknowingly or knowingly disseminating the AIDS virus. To make no efforts whatsoever to determine who is infected is to encourage further rapid AIDS spread.

Federal penalties would be imposed on physicians failing to report persons diagnosed with full-blown AIDS, intermediate AIDS or the asymptomatically infected.

6. *There must be a federal crackdown on pornography soliciting persons for high-risk sexual activities. Computerized solicitation for high-risk sexual activities and the efforts of paedophiles to seek children must be stopped.*

Society has a legitimate interest in suppressing exploitative pornography. In light of the AIDS epidemic in particular, pornography containing solicitations for sodomy and other acts responsible for AIDS transmission must be blocked. Interstate use of computers for soliciting high-risk sexual activity and for exchange of lists of children by paedophiles must be stopped.

7. *There must be a crackdown on massage parlors and vice rings promoting anonymous heterosexual promiscuity.*

AIDS spread is also fostered through establishments promoting and commercially exploiting anonymous heterosexual promiscuity. A significant number of female prostitutes have already become infected with the AIDS virus through drug abuse and bisexual males. Prostitution appears to be a major source of AIDS transmission in Africa and is a major danger for AIDS spread in the United States.

8. *Federal authorization for public and private employers to utilize AIDS risk factor questionnaires and AIDS blood screening tests in hiring. Insurance companies must be permitted to utilize these means in selecting applicants.*

Although nonsexual, nonblood transfusion-related AIDS transmission has been discounted by the CDC, other medical authorities have indicated other routes as viable means of AIDS transmission. AIDS is a lentivirus. Its incubation period is deceptively lengthy and its modes of transmission not fully understood. The genetic variability of the AIDS virus can produce dangerous changes in modes of transmission.

Researchers have already found out that AIDS is more deadly than was previously anticipated. Since AIDS is a terminal disease, it is far better to err on the side of caution now than tragically to realize later on that its capacity for spread was more potent than first contended.

Employers must have the option of refusing to hire AIDS carriers so as to protect others in the workplace. Dr. Slaff reports that General Reassurance Corporation has found the amount on all AIDS life insurance claims typically five times the average. Some states have laws prohibiting discrimination of any kind based on AIDS virus infection. Insurance companies must be able to screen out AIDS-infected individuals so as to guard against the enormous losses such as those they have already sustained in AIDS claims.

Some states and municipalities have laws prohibiting

the questioning of a prospective employee regarding his sexual behavior or orientation. These must be overridden in the interests of public safety.

9. *Sex Education in the public schools must include instruction in sound healthful principles of sexual interaction.*

A concerted effort must be made to prevent the AIDS epidemic from gaining a foothold in the nation's elementary, junior high and secondary schools.

Sex education as it is being taught in the public schools is in direct contradiction to practical guidelines to prevent AIDS. Young people are being instructed in pansexuality, the concept that all forms of sexual expression—heterosexual, bisexual, homosexual etc.—are all equally positive, healthy types of behavior. Contraceptives and birth control pills are being handed out like candy at school clinics with a simpering "play safely" for an ethical lodestar.

The do-your-own thing ethic still being taught in hygiene and sex education classes all over the country is propagating the same type of behavior which has fostered the AIDS/VD epidemics. It is utterly inconsistent with the goal of putting the brakes on AIDS transmission. Teenagers and children need to be instructed to refrain from sexual intercourse outside of marriage. They must be taught the grievous medical, personal and social consequences of heterosexual promiscuity.

Homosexuality per se must be taught as an unhealthy, unsafe and lethal sexual alternative. "It's a very major risk to enter these communities", warns June Osborn, Dean of Public Health at the University of Michigan and a professor of epidemiology. "So the fifteen or sixteen-year-old kid who's going to declare his same-sex preference should understand that there's a serious chance of infection that can truly be a matter of life and death."[14]

Summary

The shock waves of the AIDS epidemic are just beginning to be felt outside the homosexual subculture. Soon, very soon, the devastating social and economic repercussions of the epidemic will be seen and felt among all segments of society. The entire population will shudder as the anguished cries of the demented and dying rise in a ghastly crescendo. Unless drastic measures are taken to prevent the epidemic from spreading, AIDS may well become *everyone's* Final Epidemic.

What You Can Do Right Now

1. Write and/or call your Congressman:

   The Honorable _____
   U.S. House of Representatives
   Washington, D.C. 20515

   Tell him you support practical legislation to prevent AIDS spread. For example, Congressman William Dannemeyer (CA) introduced five bills aimed at halting AIDS spread:

   H.R. 3648 cuts off revenue-sharing funds to a city which permits the operation of public bathhouses if the operator knows or should know that the bath is hazardous to public health or is used for homosexual relations.

H.R. 3649 makes it a felony crime for a member of a high-risk group to donate blood.

H.R. 3646 authorizes health care professionals to utilize protective garments when caring for AIDS patients.

H.R. 3647 prohibits health care workers with AIDS from working in the health care delivery system.

H.R. Con. Res. 224 expresses the sense of Congress that public school children with AIDS should not be permitted to attend school.

Write and/or call your Congressman and ask him to cosponsor bills such as H.R. 3646, H.R. 3647, H.R. 3648, 3649, and H.R. Con. Res. 224. Ask for an investigation into why crucial facts regarding AIDS are being covered up by the national medical establishment. Tell him you want AIDS virus infection to be defined as a communicable disease under the Federal Code, section 264.
2. Write the Attorney General:

The Honorable Edwin Meese, III
Attorney General of the United States
10 Constitution Ave. NW
Washington, D.C. 20530
(202) 633-2000

Tell him you support an investigation to determine if there is collusion involved between homosexual activist groups and the national medical establishment in regards to crucial facts regarding AIDS not being released to the public. The health of our nation is at stake. Inform him that you believe the public has a right to know all the pertinent information regarding this deadly epidemic.

Tell him you support federal efforts to fight commercial sex establishments and pornography promoting AIDS spread.

If you are a medical worker or hospital patient and feel your right to personal safety has been violated by violation of proper protocol in dealing with AIDS patients, call and or write the Attorney General's Office and inform him of these violations. Persons providing such information can do so with complete confidentiality.

3. Write or call the Secretary of Education:

Mr. William J. Bennet
Secretary of Education
400 Maryland Ave. SW
Washington, D.C. 20202
(202) 426-6420

Tell him of your support for teaching sex education which promotes healthful standards of sexual conduct among the nation's young people. Explain that, especially in light of the AIDS epidemic, young persons should be discouraged from engaging in promiscuity and experimenting in pansexuality.

4. Write or call the Surgeon General:

Dr. C. Everett Koop
716G Hubert Humphrey Bldg.
200 Independence Ave. SW
Washington, D.C. 20201
(202) 245-6467

Tell him you support:
—AIDS virus infection being defined as a communicable disease under the Federal Code, section 264.
—Tuberculosis being defined as manifestation of AIDS virus infection.
—Cases of AIDS virus infection being reported to federal health authorities and contact tracing for the partners of infected individuals.

Organizations Which Can Help Persons Come out of Homosexuality

Courage
Reverend John Harvey, O.S.F.S.
P.O. Box 913
Old Chelsea
New York, NY 10113

Exodus International
P.O. Box 2121
San Rafael, CA 94912

Love in Action
P.O. Box 2655
San Rafael, CA 94912

Outpost
P.O. Box 422
Minneapolis, MN 55414

Exodus International (Europe)
Box 3
Wirral Merseyville
England L49 6NY

THE NEED FOR SOBER COMPASSION

Contempt for man and idolization of man are close neighbors. But the good man too, no less than the wicked, succumbs to the same temptation to be a despiser of mankind if he sees through all this and withdraws in disgust, leaving his fellow-men to their own devices, and if he prefers to mind his own business rather than debase himself in public life. Of course his contempt for mankind is more respectable and upright, but it is also more barren and ineffectual. . . .

But there is also an honestly intended philanthropism which amounts to the same thing as contempt for mankind. It consists in judging the man according to his latent values, according to his underlying soundness reasonableness and goodness. . . . With forced indulgence evil is interpreted as good. Baseness is overlooked and the reprehensible is excused. For one reason or another one is afraid to give a clear "no" for an answer, and one ends up by acquiescing in everything.[1]

— Dietrich Bonhoeffer.

Holistic Compassion versus Victim Identification Hysteria

One of the major purposes of this book has been to expose facts regarding AIDS which have been obscured partially or *in toto* from objective public scrutiny. Primary medical sources have been quoted verbatim with a modicum of subjective commentary. This format was intentionally designed to provide the reader with first hand information in order to permit an objective assessment of the problem. A strong exposure to solid reality, harsh as it may be, is needed in order to develop and implement effective strategies for stopping this twentieth century plague from spreading. The bulk of material in this book relates to the nature and causes of the AIDS epidemic and the enormous threat it poses to society. The objection may be raised by some that there has been insufficient space devoted to compassion and sympathy for AIDS sufferers themselves.

It should be stated outright, that persons suffering from AIDS related complex (ARC) or fulminant AIDS are truly tragic individuals. Many AIDS patients lose their minds and control of vital bodily functions as infection by the AIDS virus itself and or related brain infections progress. Their bodies become enervated and emaciated. Some go blind. Unrelenting, excruciating pain often sets in. As with those suffering from other devastating terminal illnesses, those who survive somewhat longer than average may not consider themselves among the more fortunate.

As their symptoms become more pronounced, AIDS patients become unable to perform their job tasks adequately. Although private or public sources of disability income may be available, other expenses, especially medical, frequently render this reduced level of income insufficient. Unemployed and with a limited source of disability income, personal savings become rapidly depleted.

In addition, AIDS patients are sometimes shunned by their friends, families, loved ones and others. Severely ill and infectious, in financial straits, cut off from their emotional support systems and facing the prospect of imminent AIDS death, AIDS sufferers may be said to constitute the Untouchables of Western society. Their plight evokes profound pathos in anyone with a measure of human sensitivity and kindness. Dr. Restak rightfully points out that persons with AIDS "should be treated with the care and compassion due to anyone who is ill with a so-far incurable and invariably fatal disease". Intensive research toward finding a cure and vaccine must continue, no matter how arduous and impossible the task may seem.

The exigency of providing compassionate care for terminally ill AIDS patients should not, however, be permitted to override the necessity of realistically evaluating the major factors fostering the epidemic and developing effective means of halting the spread of contagion. True compassion regarding the AIDS epidemic must be holistic in scope. It must encompass a sympathetic concern for protecting *society as a whole* from acquiring the disease from those presently infected. In the pell mell rush to identify with the plight of AIDS sufferers, compassionate concern for the rest of society has been largely ignored. Permeated with heterophobia, AIDS victim identification hysteria has dangerously impeded compassionate steps being taken to safeguard the health of the rest of society.

Along with AIDS sufferers, chain-smoking lung cancer or emphysema patients should receive compassionate treatment and care as well. Minimizing or downplaying the harmful effects of smoking in order not to disconcert those dying or still engaging in the behavior at risk would be patently dishonest and irresponsible. On the contrary, the Surgeon General along with many medical groups has been quite vocal in stating that smoking causes a variety of grave diseases. An increasing number of private businesses (offices, restaurants etc.) and municipalities have enacted regulations prohibiting smoking in various areas to protect others from the harmful effects of second-hand smoke.

Out of a compassionate humanitarian concern for those who would otherwise have their lives snuffed out by drunk drivers, many states have enacted increasingly stiff penalties for those who drive while impaired by alcohol. The high incidence of teenagers involved in drunk driving accidents along with other social factors has caused the legal drinking age to be raised to twenty-one in many areas.

The overwhelming majority of those infected with AIDS in the United States thus far are male homosexuals who have repeatedly engaged in grossly insanitary, pathological behaviors utterly inconducive to human health and at grave risk of spreading a host of highly infectious diseases. This crucial factor should not be minimized or glossed over as incidental.

However, the response of homosexual activists and their sympathetic allies in the media and elsewhere to the AIDS crisis has revealed an ideological mindset which has become so ingrained that it will not or cannot face biological reality. In the face of lethal pandemics correlated with homosexual acts and behavior patterns, every effort is being made to ensure the continued growth of the subculture after their present ranks are utterly depleted due to disease. In a frenetic effort to preserve the notion of homosexuality as a healthy alternative lifestyle, legal mechanisms have been and are being put in place to block any practical efforts to prevent AIDS from spreading throughout the entire population. In the interests of compassion for those not yet infected, every effort must be made to proscribe legally those already infected with the AIDS virus from spreading the infection to the rest of the population.

Notwithstanding the *ex cathedra* promulgations of the American psychological and psychiatric associations to the contrary, true compassion and intellectual honesty demands admitting that the entire homosexual liberation movement has been a form of biological mass suicide. The Pied Pipers of the homosexual liberation movement have led hundreds of thousands, perhaps millions of young bathhouse habitués to an impending AIDS death. Redolent of the mass carnage induced by bisexual demagogue Jim Jones in Guyana, they have promised their followers nirvana and have led them instead into the abyss of depravity and despair.

Tragically, many of their devotees still parade about, disease riddled and dying, unabashedly promoting acceptance of the very behavior leading to their ruin. Their benighted sympathetic allies in the media and elsewhere march alongside them, holding fund-raising banquets for AIDS research. Oddly enough, Hollywood's finest have not seen fit to hold black tie fund-raising affairs for research on herpes, chlamydia or the new highly resistant strains of gonorrhea. The media has also been conspicuously silent regarding deadly Delta hepatitis which is now spreading among non-drug abusing members of the homosexual subculture as a result of continued promiscuous sodomy and other pathological behaviors.

Lest this indictment of recalcitrant homosexual activism seem somewhat overstated, picture a parade of thousands of emaciated, terminally ill lung cancer and emphysema patients marching down the street chain smoking carrying large banners emblazoned with the slogan, "Fighting for Our Lives" and angrily blaming the government for not finding a cure or vaccine for their respective self-induced diseases. The National *Happy* Chain Smokers/Lung Cancer Victims Task Force is formed, demanding an end to stereotyping smokers as hacking, wheezing individuals with a high rate of lethal heart and lung diseases. They point out that emphysema and lung cancer are not solely smokers' diseases. Stridently and militantly, they hoarsely demand a stop to smokerphobia and sagely propound the wisdom of safe smoking techniques. The major networks begin running show after show on lung cancer and emphysema patients who never smoked. Smokers, it is widely contended, should not be stigmatized and discriminated against on the basis of their air inhalation orientation. A person's individual preference for inhaling voluminous quantities of smoke filled with tar, nicotine and other carcinogens is protected by the constitutional right to privacy. After all, who's to say whether cigarette smoking is right or wrong?

As incongruous as the above scenario appears, it accurately portrays the grotesque parody of honest compassion for AIDS sufferers and potential victims that homosexual activists and their allies have demonstrated in response to the AIDS epidemic ravaging their numbers and others. The slogan "Fighting for Our Lives" can be translated from the gayspeak, "Fighting for the right to continue engaging in the gamut of pernicious homosexual perversion without suffering the medical consequences." A compassion for AIDS sufferers which does not include a resounding *caveat emptor* regarding any involvement in the homosexual subculture is nothing more than a mawkish hysteria which impedes effective steps at preventing the epidemic from spreading.

The promotion of "safe" techniques of homosexual perversion by homosexual leaders and their bedfellows in the media, medical and educational establishments is a fraudulent myth which will prove damning to the homosexual subculture in general along with those who are newly proselyted into their group. If the proof of the pudding is in the eating, than those sampling the desserts of homosexual perversion must be honestly told to expect to receive its inherent biological deserts; bodily trauma, parasites, venereal disease, liver disorders and a nightmarish death from AIDS. True compassion demands integrity in informing those who would otherwise perish of the real dangers connected with homosexual acts.

Non-Moralizing: The Sin of Omission

Jewish and Christian Biblical safe-sex guidelines and AIDS prevention:

Whenever we break with moral tradition we do so at our own risk. . . . [2]
    — John C. Fletcher, Ph.D Assistant for Bioethics at the National Institutes of Health

The AIDS virus may well take the joy out of lustful anonymous sex and replace it with a manic, desperate, self-destructive quality. [3]
    — Dr. James Slaff, Medical Investigator, the National Institutes of Health

There is a syllogism pervading the response of the media, educational and medical, establishments to the AIDS crisis. According to their line of reasoning, the social and sexual mores which developed prior to AIDS were positive and liberating for all those involved, homosexual and heterosexual alike. In no way should it be intimated that any type of pre-AIDS sexual behavior was inappropriate or wrong. The remote suggestion that some forms of sexual expression would have been better off discouraged and avoided in the first place is branded as unfair and unloving. Interjecting any concept of sexual morality into solutions for preventing the spread of AIDS is seen as a cardinal sin. AIDS, it is argued, is merely an incidental biological party spoiler. If it were not for the worrisome possibility of personal and societal self-extinction, everyone could have continued wallowing in libertinism and perversion *ad infinitum ad 'nauseum* without negative consequences. An article in *Life* states: "Public education about AIDS has scarcely begun. Some experts are calling for a massive campaign to warn sexually active young people to take precautions—such as using condoms—against the disease." The fear of catching AIDS, the writer grimly predicts, could cause virginity and abstinence to come back in vogue thus making "late twentieth century America an *anxious* and altered society."[4]

There is a fundamental premise lacking in the effete get-to-know-your-partners-first and crank out the condoms response to the AIDS and venereal disease epidemics. It is the glaring reality that the lax sexual mores of Western culture have proven destructive to the social fabric of civilization, apart from any of the infectious diseases accompanying promiscuity.

Harvard therapist, Dr. Armand Nicoli, commenting on the encroaching trends of sexual liberation as far back as 1965 aptly noted:

This is what a psychiatrist sees—unwanted pregnancies, ill-advised marriages, abortions followed by severe depressions and haunting repetitive nightmares, disillusionment, frustration, despondency, suicide. It is for this reason that psychiatrists are concerned about this happening. It is for this reason that many of them are concerned that something is wrong somewhere.

This new sexual freedom is not what people are led to believe. . . . It certainly does not lead to prolonged ecstatic pleasure. There is no evidence that it leads to greater freedom and openness and more meaningful relationships between the sexes. Quite the opposite. And there is certainly little evidence that it leads to exhilarating relief from stifling inihibitions. When you focus on what this new freedom really entails, one can't but be impressed that it doesn't appear to be much fun. . . . Somehow there has been a great deal of deception going on. Somehow a lot of people have been *deluded.*[5] [Italics theirs].

Reflecting on the advanced decline of the traditional family unit and the dramatic rise in broken homes, liberal columnist Carl Rowan belatedly mused in the May 28, 1985, issue of the Washington Post:

I read a Census Bureau report the other day and found myself wishing that we had armies of people telling our teenagers that they ought to shun sex and childbirth out of wedlock, and that they ought to take marriage as a serious, longlasting commitment. . . .

These figures on one-parent families tell us a lot about the social malaise of modern America—the vanishing sexual, moral, social and legal taboos without which Americans have produced drastic increases in divorces, desertions, and children born out of wedlock. . . . These figures also tell us a lot about the social ills—crime, ignorance, sickness—that future generations must deal with because so many children now face so much neglect and need.[6]

Research indicates that 400,000 to 500,000 adolescents in the United States attempt suicide annually. Dr. Pamela Cantor, president of the American Association of Suicidology states: "The breakup of the family unit, increased family violence and rootlessness are contributing factors."[7]

It must also be realized that fear of contracting AIDS alone will not provide a sufficient impetus for many people to alter their sexual behavior patterns. As the late Archbishop Fulton J. Sheen stated:

> I think one of the reasons for promiscuity today is the absence of purpose in life. When we are driving a car and become lost, we generally drive faster; so when there is an absence of the full meaning of life, there is a tendency to compensate for it by speed, drugs, and intensity of feeling.[8]

Dr. David Mace has written:

> Sex must be the servant of love, of parenthood, of home life. A sound code of sexual behavior, therefore, is one which leads to a state of society in which marriage and family living are happy and wholesome, stable and secure. . . .
>
> What we need is a new idea of chastity, as a discipline gladly accepted so that human love can be kept warm and tender and unsullied. This idea of chastity means refusing to use sex at subhuman levels and for selfish and antisocial ends. It is not the renunciation of sexual love as something evil. Rather it is the recognition that sexual love is something too good to be spoiled by misuse.[9]

It may be begging the question, but it needs to be asked.

Is society really better off with:
— a 60% divorce rate
— 1,500,000 abortions annually
— 400,000 pregnancies out of wedlock annually
— 20,000,000 to 30,000,000 cases of incurable genital
  herpes
— paedophilia, incest and teenage prostitution at epidemic levels
— 3,000,000 new cases of chlamydia annually
— 3,000,000 new cases of gonorrhea
— 1,000,000 cases of pelvic inflammatory disease (PID)
— 100,000s of adolescent girls and women permanently
  sterilized as a result of gonorrhea-induced PID
— 10,000s of women having developed cervical cancer
  as a result of promiscuity, herpes and venereal warts
— millions of young men facing a prospect of AIDS
  death through involvement in homosexuality.

Or perhaps, just perhaps, the millenia-old Jewish and
Christian Biblical guidelines have been relevant all along.
Bestiality, homosexuality, incest, fornication and adultery are all explicitly proscribed in the Scriptures.[10]
Some critics, notably those holding to homosexual liberation theology, contend that since many dietary restrictions are generally no longer observed by contemporary
Jews (with the exception of Orthodox and Conservative
groups) and by the Christian Church, Old Testament
laws forbidding homosexual acts should also be seen as
no longer relevant. Regulations regarding diet, animal
sacrifices and performance of religious rituals in the
temple were part of the ceremonial law. The ceremonial law was designed to cultivate reverence for the
holiness of God and in the Christian view to point the
way to the coming Messiah. Christians believe that
since Christ is the promised Messiah, adherence to

ceremonial observances is no longer required. According to the New Testament, Christ did not abolish the moral law. He articulated its radical demand for inward as well as outward obedience more fully (e.g., Mt 5:17-20). It should be noted that the prohibition against male homosexual perversion in Leviticus is stated in the same section with injunctions against incest, adultery, bestiality and infant sacrifice. Commandments forbidding such behavior are part of the unchanging moral Law of God. According to both the Torah and New Testament Scriptures, the divine moral Law is still in effect. (For a more comprehensive treatment of the Scriptural passages regarding homosexuality the reader is referred to *Homosexuality: A Biblical View,* Greg L. Bahnsen [Baker Book House Company, 1978], pp. 27-61.)

Orthodox and traditional Jews and Christians and other persons with a high regard for the monogamous, married, heterosexual family unit have no need to apologize for attempting to inject a healthy dose of moral rectitude into the AIDS crisis. They should not be cowed by the supercilious derision of homosexual activists and their sympathizers crying foul for "using" AIDS to promote traditional sexual morality.

It is the self-appointed prophets of nihilism and pansexual libertinism who have succeeded in fostering the conditions leading to the biological and social downfall of society. They are the ones who aggressively sought to get the courts to sanction the growth of the bars, clubs and bathhouses which have been prime breeding grounds for AIDS contagion. They are the ones who have propagated the specious image of homosexuality being "gay" knowing full well that pandemics of virulent diseases were running rife. They are the ones *still* contemptuously insisting that homosexuality be taught in graphic detail as a healthy alternative form of sexual expression in the nation's elementary and secondary school hygiene classes. With AIDS, the horrendous physiological consequences of their deathstyle can no longer be concealed. Chagrined by this unassailable medical contraindication, they are venting their wrath on those who have been affirming the wisdom of traditional Biblical morality all along.

Christians and other citizens of good will have been affirming for years prior to the onset of AIDS that legal and social acceptance of homosexuality is contrary to the public good. Truly effective safe sex guidelines were in place long before the AIDS and venereal disease epidemics provoked the hedonist crowd into coming up with the idea that homosexual acts and heterosexual promiscuity might not be the ideal alternative life styles they had extolled.

It is time for people to realize that society stands on the brink of an imminent self-induced AIDS holocaust. Pecksniffian advisories on therapeutic techniques of perversion and promiscuity are a base deception. Saccharine platitudes about pansexual "serial monogamy" (coupling with only one partner for weeks or months at a time) are intellectually dishonest. With two million or more persons already infected with the AIDS virus, a little promiscuity will go a long way toward spreading mass contagion.

Only those who intransigently abide by Biblical standards of sexual morality will be able to guard themselves effectively against sexually transmitted AIDS virus infection. Avoidance of homosexual behavior, abstinence before marriage and fidelity afterwards are the only truly reliable means of safe sexual interaction.

Unfortunately, there are situations where a person

who has been abiding by these principles becomes engaged to someone who has not, and the other person is knowingly or unknowingly infected with the AIDS virus. As Dr. George Lundberg, editor of the *Journal of the American Medical Association,* has recommended, pre-marital AIDS blood screening tests ought to be considered as a preventive in this regard.

Persons wishing compassionately to share their religious faith with those in the primary risk group for AIDS must realize they do them no service by trying to excuse away promiscuity and homosexual perversion as benign pecadilloes. Dr. J. L. Fletcher, one of the few in the medical profession with the intellectual candor and personal courage squarely to address the correlation between abandonment of traditional moral views regarding homosexuality and the rise of AIDS has editorialized:

> If we act as empirical scientists, can we not see the implications of the data before us? If homosexuality, or even just male homosexuality is "OK", then why the high prevalence of associated complications both in general and especially in regard to AIDS? Might not these "complications" be "consequences"? Might it not be that our society's approval of homosexuality is an error and that the unsubtle words of the Bible are frightfully correct? . . .
>
> From an empirical medical standpoint alone, current scientific observation seems to require the conclusion that homosexuality is a pathological condition. . . . Certain cause and effect data are convincing—so convincing that health care providers in this age of unbridled enthusiasm for preventive medicine would do well to seek reversal treatment for their homosexual patients just as vigorously as they would for alcoholics or heavy cigarette smokers, for what may not be treated might well be avoided.[11]

Dr. Fletcher's advice should be heeded by all persons counseling present and potential high risk group members regarding new or continued involvement in the Stygian milieu of the homosexual subculture.

APPENDIX A

A LETTER TO THE EDITOR

... not everyone infected with the AIDS virus will progress to CDC-defined AIDS.

It is true that acquired immune deficiency syndrome, as originally, narrowly, defined by CDC for the limited purpose of epidemiological analysis of a new disease phenomenon, required either a life-threatening opportunistic infection moderately indicative of profound immune deficiency, or Kaposi's sarcoma, as a prerequisite for the diagnosis of AIDS. However, now that it is clear that CDC-defined AIDS is only one or two facets of a highly specific, viral disease, spreading for the first time ever as an epidemic in man, the decision by CDC, on 28 June 1985, to retain this definition with only trivial modifications[1] is a bureaucratic decision by officials which obscures the full range of the biological interaction between the AIDS virus and man. As the epidemic evolves it is becoming ever more apparent that the immune deficiency aspect of AIDS may turn out to be only a relatively unimportant part of the disease caused by infection with the AIDS virus. Certainly, Kaposi's sarcoma is only a rare complication of AIDS virus infection, largely confined to homosexual men.

Just as the term AIDS misleads, because it diverts attention exclusively to the immune deficiency sometimes seen with AIDS virus infection, so the attempt to name the virus 'Human T-cell lymphotropic virus type III' is also misleading. HTLV-III is a different virus from HTLV-I and HTLV-II, both genetically and in its pathogenesis and transmission. Furthermore, it focuses attention on the relatively unimportant lymphotropism of the virus, and obscures its far more deadly neurotropic and pneumotropic properties.

The neurotropic properties of the AIDS virus are now well known to clinicians caring for patients dying from AIDS, though little has been published on this subject. It had been assumed that progressive dementia and cerebral atrophy, which so commonly precedes death, were caused by opportunistic viruses such as cytomegalovirus, herpes simplex or polyomavirus, whereas it is the AIDS virus itself which is directly destroying the brain. As the AIDS epidemic progresses, AIDS-virus encephalopathy may become the major cause of death, but unless these patients have an irrelevant opportunistic infection they will not be regarded as having CDC-defined AIDS.

The pneumotropic properties of the AIDS virus are less well known. However, chronic lymphoid interstitial pneumonitis (CLIP) is such a characteristic feature of paediatric AIDS that CDC, when it redefined AIDS on 28 June 1985, decided to include CLIP. Serological tests for HTLV-111/LAV antibodies had to be positive, but no evidence of opportunistic infections was required for the diagnosis, provided that it occurred in children under the age of thirteen[1]. Evidence now emerging from Central Africa shows that in the later stages of the AIDS epidemic, large numbers of adults as well as children develop CLIP, often in association with pulmonary tuberculosis.

Pulmonary tuberculosis, combined with pulmonary AIDS, would be highly lethal because both the microbes would be coughed into the air, and both remain infectious for more than a week at room temperature[2]. It is unlikely that CDC will classify such cases as AIDS for fear of causing public hysteria; and also because this would conflict with their favourite hypothesis that AIDS is a venereal disease.

J. Seale
Former Consultant in Venereology, the Middlesex and St. Thomas' Hospitals, London (reprinted from the *Journal of the Royal Society of Medicine,* 77[1986]:121)

APPENDIX B

AIDS:
THE IMPERATIVE FOR DISCIPLINE

Now everyone in the country knows what AIDS (acquired immune deficiency syndrome) is—a viral disease that is incurable, inexorably fatal. The only sure means of prevention is a single-partner life style and the ability to avoid infected blood transfusions and used hypodermic needles. The victims so far have principally been homosexuals, but the disease is spreading to a wider population.

According to the media, the public has gotten into a state of panic about AIDS. If this is so, it is unnecessary, but the degree to which it is unnecessary depends on where society goes from here. AIDS is really quite easily preventable, and for society as a whole it could soon be put into decline. However, in simply reading these facts, some who feel their own personal sexual philosophy threatened will scream "intolerance", "homophobia" and even "sexual McCarthyism".

California Congressman Henry Waxman and others are calling for something like a Manhattan Project to find preventions and cures. However, the fact is that simple, relatively inexpensive public health measures could cause AIDS to virtually disappear over time. Applied individually, they will work individually, but applied collectively they could kiss this epidemic goodbye. As one virologist at the National Institutes of Health told me when he heard I was writing this article, "Get the point across about life style; if a sufficient number of gays, promiscuous heterosexuals and IV drug users were able to change that, this disease would go into decline. Tell the transmitters what a heavy burden they have on their shoulders for humanity."

The public health measures? Single-partner life style; no promiscuity; screening of the national blood supply (though some cases will always slip through, since serum antibodies may not appear for up to six months after exposure). The difficulty here is that public health and public morals (traditional variety) are analogous to two concentric circles.

Perhaps for this reason, even some public health officials with serious responsibility for the control of the spread of AIDS are acting peculiarly. Such a one is the Dallas Health Department county epidemiologist, with whom I discussed the epidemiologically obvious need to close down the Club Dallas bathhouse. (This establishment, with a reported patronage of over 30,000, has recently been advertising special cheap locker rates for teenagers.) At first he said he was unaware the club was still open, then defended such clubs (it would be "purely political" to close them down).

Despite the prevalence of some benighted "health" officials, I believe it would be worth mounting a Manhattan Project aimed at effecting life-style change. I think most people do. In any event, if one sees the urgent needs of the moment in a predominantly moral light, such a posture would be hypocritical if it did not also include compassion for, and willingness to contribute to, the serious needs of *all* AIDS sufferers.

Dr. Gordon Muir
Executive with a major pharmaceutical company. Reprinted from *Texas Business* (December 16, 1985).

NOTES

Introduction
The Dangers Are Real

1. J. Seale, "AIDS Virus Infection: Prognosis and Transmission", *J Roy Soc Med* 1985;78:613-615.

2. J. W. Curran, "The Epidemiology and Prevention of the Acquired Immunodeficiency Syndrome", *Ann of Int Med* 1985;103:657-662.

3. Ibid., p. 658.

4. J. I. Slaff and J. K. Brubaker, *The AIDS Epidemic: How You Can Protect Yourself and Your Family — Why You Must* (New York: Warner Books, 1985), pp. 159-160. S. L. Sivak and G. P. Wormer, "How Common Is HTLV-III Infection in the United States?", *N Eng J Med* 1985;313:1352. J. Adler, N. F. Greenberg et al., "The AIDS Conflict", *Newsweek*, 23 September 1985, p. 18.

Chapter 1
Design for Disaster — How the AIDS Virus Operates

1. *Fort Worth Star-Telegram*, 30 July 1985.

2. R. C. Gallo and F. Wong-Staal, "A Human T-Lymphotropic Retrovirus (HTLV-III) as the Cause of the Acquired Immunodeficiency Syndrome", *Ann of Int Med* 1985;103:679-689. P. J. Kanki et al., "Antibodies to Simian T-Lymphotropic Retrovirus Type III in African Green Monkeys and Recognition of STLV-III Viral Proteins by AIDS and Related Sera", *Lancet*, 8 June 1985, p. 1330-1332. M. Essex et al., "Antigens of Human T-Lymphotropic Virus Type III/Lymphadenopathy-Associated Virus", *Ann of Int Med* 1985; 103:700-703.

3. Slaff and Brubaker, *The AIDS Epidemic* (New York: Warner Books, 1985), p. 112.

4. F. P. Siegal and M. Siegal, *AIDS: The Medical Mystery* (New York: Grove Press, 1983), p. 119. Slaff and Brubaker, op. cit., p. 182.

5. Acquired Immune Deficiency Syndrome (AIDS): Precautions for Clinical and Laboratory Staffs, *MMWR,* 5 November 1982. D. Peter Drotman (CDC), "Insect Borne Transmission of AIDS?" *JAMA* 1985;254:1085.

6. Seale, "AIDS Virus Infection: Prognosis and Transmission", *JRSM* 1985;78:615.

7. "Follow-Up on Kaposi's Sarcoma and Pneumocystis Pneumonia", *MMWR,* 28 August 1981.

8. "Persistent Generalized Lymphadenopathy among Homosexual Males", *MMWR* 1982;31:365.

9. Jeanne Kassler, *Gay Men's Health: A Guide to the AID Syndrome and Other Sexually Transmitted Diseases* (New York: Harper and Row, 1983).

10. "Follow-up on Kaposi's Sarcoma and Pneumocystis Pneumonia", *MMWR,* 28 August 1981.

11. David A. Noebel, *The Homosexual Revolution* (Manitou Springs, Col.: Summit Press, 1985), p. 85.

12. F. P. Siegal and M. Siegal, op. cit., p. 68-103.

13. P. Piot et al., "Acquired Immunodeficiency Syndrome in a Heterosexual Population in Zaire", *Lancet,* 14 July 1984, p. 68.

14. K. M. De Cock, "AIDS: An Old Disease from Africa?" *British Medical Journal* 1984;289:306-308. "Update: Acquired Immune Deficiency Syndrome (AIDS)—United States", *MMWR* 1984; 33:357-9.

15. "Update: Acquired Immunodeficiency Syndrome—Europe", *MMWR,* 2 November 1984, pp. 607-609.

16. G. B. Scott et al., "Mothers of Infants with the Acquired Immune Deficiency Syndrome: Evidence for Both Symptomatic and Asymptomatic Carriers", *JAMA* 1985;253:363-366. G. B. Scott et al., "Acquired Immunodeficiency in Infants", *N Eng J Med* 1984;310:76-81.

17. G. M. Shearer, "Other factors to Consider in Infantile AIDS", *N Eng J Med* 1984;311:189-190.

18. S. Broder and R. C. Gallo, "A Pathogenic Retrovirus (HTLV-III) Linked to AIDS", *N Eng J Med* 1984;311:1292-1297.

19. *Fort Worth Star-Telegram,* 30 July 1985.

20. L. Montagnier, "Lymphadenopathy-Associated Virus: From Molecular Biology to Pathogenicity", *Ann of Int Med* 1985;103: 689-693.

21. J. B. Brunet and R. A. Ancelle, "The International Occurrence of the Acquired Immunodeficiency Syndrome", *Ann of Int Med* 1985;103:673, citing A. K. Kapend, W. Odio, "La cryptococcose neuromeningee", *NJANJA Med* 1983;6:17-21 and B. Lamey and N. Melameka, "Aspects cliniques et epidemiologiques de la cryptococcose a Kinasha", *Med Trop* 1982;42:507-11.

22. Seale, op. cit., p. 615.

23. W. A. Blattner et al., "Epidemiology of Human T-Lymphotropic Virus Type III and the Risk of Acquired Immunodeficiency Syndrome", *Ann of Int Med* 1985;103:665-670.

24. J. A. Levy et al., "Infection by the Retrovirus Associated with the Acquired Immunodeficiency Syndrome; Clinical, Biological and Molecular Features", *Ann of Int Med* 1985;103:694-699. L. S. Fujikawa et al., "Isolation of Human T-Lymphotropic Virus Type III from Tears of a Patient with the Acquired Immunodeficiency Syndrome", *Lancet* 1985;2:529.

25. M. W. Vogt et al., "Isolation of HTLV–III/LAV from Cervical Secretions of Women at Risk for AIDS", *Lancet* 1986;1:525–527. C. B. Wopsy et al., "Isolation of AIDS–Associated Virus from Genital Secretions of Women with Antibodies to the Virus", *Lancet* 1986;1:527–529.

26. J. Laurence, "The Immune System in AIDS", *Scientific American* 1985;253:84–93.

27. J. Laurence, "Keeping Cool about AIDS", *Dallas Morning News,* 7 October 1985.

28. J. H. Tanne, "The Last Word on Avoiding AIDS", *New York Magazine,* 7 October 1985, p. 29.

29. J. Seale, op. cit., p. 614.

30. G. M. Shaw et al., "HTLV–III Infection in Brains of Children and Adults with AIDS Encephalopathy", *Science* 1985;227:177–182.

31. C. A. Rosen et al., "The Location of Cis-Acting Regulatory Sequences in the Human T-Cell Lymphotropic Virus Type III (HTLV–III/LAV) Long Terminal Repeat", *Cell* 1985;41:813–823.

32. Gallo and Wong-Staal, op. cit., p. 685.

33. F. P. Siegal, International Conference on AIDS, 14–17 April 1985, Atlanta, CDC/WHO, cited in J. Seale, "AIDS Virus Infection: Prognosis and Transmission", *J Roy Soc Med* 1985;75:614.

34. D. Armstrong et al., "Treatment of Infections in Patients with the Acquired Immunodeficiency Syndrome", *Ann of Int Med* 1985; 103:738–741.

35. Slaff and Brubaker, op. cit. p. 140.

36. K. Tenner-Racz et al., "Altered Follicular Dendritic Cells and Virus-Like Particles in AIDS and AIDS–Related Lymphadenopathy", *Lancet,* 12 January 1985.

37. D. D. Ho et al., "HTLV-III in the Semen and Blood of a Healthy Homosexual Man", *Science* 1984;226:451.

38. Slaff and Brubaker, op. cit., p. 28.

39. R. C. Gallo and Wong-Staal, op. cit., p. 679.

40. D. Gelman et al., "AIDS", *Newsweek,* 12 August 1985, p. 22.

41. Joel L. Nitzkin, M.D., and Mark J. Merkens, M.D., Monroe County Department of Health, Rochester, NY, letter to the editor *JAMA* 1985;253:3398, citing draft federal regulations in the *MMWR* 1985;34:1-5.

42. J. Curran, "The Epidemiology and Prevention of the Acquired Immunodeficiency Syndrome", *Ann of Int Med* 1985;103:660.

43. Slaff and Brubaker, op. cit., pp. 31 and 140.

44. W. A. Blattner et al., op. cit., pp. 665-670. G. B. Scott, "Mothers of Infants with Acquired Immunodeficiency Syndrome (AIDS): Evidence for Both Symptomatic and Asymptomatic Carriers", *JAMA* 1985;253:363-366.

45. M. H. Heckler, "The Challenge of the Acquired Immunodeficiency Syndrome", *Ann of Int Med* 1985;103:655-656.

46. J. W. Curran, op. cit., p. 658.

47. Slaff and Brubaker, op. cit., p. 142.

48. Ibid.

49. C. S. Thomas et al., "HTLV-III and Psychiatric Disturbance", *Lancet,* 17 August 1985, pp. 395-396.

50. Seale, op. cit., p. 614.

51. Slaff and Brubaker, op. cit., p. 125.

52. J. Kassler, *Gay Men's Health: A Guide to the AIDS Syndrome and Other Sexually Transmitted Diseases* (New York: Harper & Row, 1983), pp. 1-36.

53. Acquired Immunodeficiency Syndrome (AIDS) Weekly Surveillance Report, United States AIDS Activity Center for Infectious Diseases, Center for Disease Control, 14 January 1985.

54. Siegal and Siegal, op. cit., p. 2.

55. R. Soave and P. Ma, "Cryptosporidiosis", *Arch Intern Med* 1985;145:70-72.

56. S. B. Kalish et al., "Diagnosis and Treatment of Acquired Immune Deficiency States and Opportunistic Infections", in D. Ostrow et al., *Sexually Transmitted Diseases in Homosexual Men* (New York: Plenum Medical Book Company, 1983), p. 221.

57. D. Greenspan et al., "Oral 'Hairy' Leukoplakia in Male Homosexuals: Evidence of Association with Both Papillomavirus and a Herpes-Group Virus", *Lancet,* 13 October 1984, pp. 831-834.

58. "Leads from the MMWR—Oral Viral Lesion (Hairy Leukoplakia) Associated with Acquired Immunodeficiency Syndrome", *JAMA* 1985;254;1694.

59. A. M. Levine et al., "Retrovirus and Malignant Lymphoma in Homosexual Men", *JAMA* 1985;254:1921-1925.

60. A. M. Levine et al., "B-Cell Lymphoma in Two Monogamous Homosexual Men", *Arch Intern Med* 1985;145:479-481.

61. *Lancet,* 25 January 1986, p. 193.

62. M. Cimons, "TB Could Serve as Early Warning against AIDS", *Dallas Times Herald,* 28 November 1985.

63. M. A. Fischl et al., "Tuberculosis Brain Abscesses and Toxoplasma Encephalitis in a Patient with the Acquired Immunodeficiency Syndrome", *JAMA* 1985;253:3428-3430.

64. *JAMA* 1984;252:2038.

65. "Economic impact of AIDS shown", *Fort Worth Star-Telegram,* 10 January 1986.

66. J. Seale, op. cit., p. 614.

67. G. M. Shaw et al., op. cit., 177-182.

68. Gallo and Wong-Staal, op. cit., pp. 680-681.

69. L. Montagnier, op. cit., p. 691.

70. Seale, op. cit., p. 613.

71. *Time,* 12 August 1985, p. 41.

72. W. A. Blattner et al., op. cit., pp. 665-670.

73. J. Levy et al., op. cit., citing B. R. Sigurdsson, "A Chronic Encephalitis of Sheep: with general remarks on infections which develop slowly and some of their special characteristics", *Br Vet J* 1954;110:341-354 and A. T. Haase, "The Slow Infection Caused by Visna Virus", *Curr Top Microbiol Immunol* 1975;72:101-56.

74. Seale, op. cit., p. 614.

75. Slaff and Brubaker, op. cit., p. 171.

76. Seale, op. cit., p. 614.

77. Slaff and Brubaker, op. cit., p. 173.

78. Ibid., p. 260.

79. R.-M. E. Fincher, "AIDS-Related Complex in a Heterosexual Man Seven Weeks after a Transfusion", *N Eng J Med* 1985;313: 1226-1227.

80. D. P. Francis et al., "The Natural History of Infection with the

Lymphadenopathy-Associated Virus Human T-Lymphotropic Virus Type III", *Ann of Int Med* 1985;103:721.

81. Seale, op. cit., p. 614.

82. Slaff and Brubaker, op. cit., pp. 173-174.5.

83. Seale, op. cit., p. 615.

Chapter 2
How the Epidemic Has Spread

1. *The Advocate*, 28 May, 1985, p. 33.

2. "Update: Acquired Immunodeficiency—Europe," *MMWR*, 18 January 1984, p. 29.

3. J. J. Goedert et al., "Determinants of Retrovirus (HTLV–III) Antibody and Immunodeficiency Conditions in Homosexual Men", *Lancet*, 29 September 1984, pp. 711-715.

4. David G. Ostrow, Terri A. Sandholzer and Yehudi M. Felman, *Sexually Transmitted Diseases in Homosexual Men* (New York: Plenum Medical Book Co., 1983), pp. 141-149.

5. Pearl Ma and Donald Armstrong, *The Acquired Immune Deficiency Syndrome and Infections of Homosexual Men* (New York: Yorke Medical Books, 1984), p. 4.

6. Ostrow et al., op. cit., p. 144.

7. A. Bernal et al., "Endoscopic and Pathologic Features of Gastrointestinal Kaposi's Sarcoma: A Report of Four Cases in Patients with the Acquired Immune Deficiency Syndrome", *Gastrointestinal Endoscopy* 1985;31:74-77.

8. Ostrow et al., op. cit., p. 192.

9. H. W. Jaffe et al., "National Case-Control Study of Kaposi's Sarcoma and Pneumocystis Carinii Pneumonia in Homosexual Men: part 2, Laboratory Results", *Ann of Int Med* 1983;99:145-151.

10. J. J. Goedert, op. cit., pp. 711-715.

11. G. M. Mavligit et al., "Chronic Immune Stimulation by Sperm Alloantigens; Support for the Hypothesis That Spermatozoa Induce Immune Dysregulation in Homosexual Males", *JAMA* 1984;251: 237-241.

12. *Science,* 27 April 1984.

13. S. Hsia et al., "Unregulated Production of Virus and/or Sperm Specific Anti-Idiotypic Antibodies as a Cause of AIDS", *Lancet,* 2 June 1984, pp. 1212-1214.

14. Mavligit, op. cit., pp. 237-241.

15. Ibid., pp. 240-241.

16. D. J. Anderson and E. J. Yunis, " 'Trojan horse' Leukocytes in AIDS", *N Eng J Med* 1983;309:984-985, cited in "The Acquired Immunodeficiency Syndrome: Commentary-Council on Scientific Affairs", *JAMA* 1984;252:2037-2043.

17. Mavligit, op. cit., p. 241.

18. J. M. Richards et al., "Rectal Insemination Modifies Immune Responses in Rabbits", *Science* 1984;224:390-392. U. Hurtenbach and G. M. Shearer, "Germ cell-induced immune suppression in mice: Effect of synergeneic spermatozoa on cell-mediated immune responses", *J Exp Med* 1982;155:1719-1729.

19. Mavligit, op. cit., p. 241.

20. Ma and Armstrong, op. cit., p. 415.

21. Goedert et al., op. cit., 711-715.

216   THE AIDS COVER-UP?

22. A. P. Bell and M. S. Weinberg, *Homosexualities: A Study of Diversity among Men and Women* (New York: Simon & Schuster, 1978), pp. 106-109.

23. Ostrow, op. cit., pp. 151-156.

24. Jaffe et al., "The Acquired Immunodeficiency Syndrome in Gay Men", *Ann of Int Med* 1985;103:662-640.

25. D. J. Atkinson, *Homosexuals in the Christian Fellowship* (Michigan: W. B. Eerdmans, 1979), p. 48.

26. Enrique T. Rueda, *The Homosexual Network* (Old Greenwich, Con.: Devin Adair, 1982), p. 89 citing *The Journal* (Manitou Springs, Col.), June 1, 1981; the *Sacramento Bee* (Sacramento, Calif.), 13 March 1981.

27. Ostrow, op. cit., p. 189.

28. "GMHC Revises Risk-Reduction Guidelines for Healthier Sex", *New York Native,* 21-27 October 1985, p. 59.

29. Rueda, op. cit., p 38.

30. P. K. Lewin, *Can Med Assoc J* 1985;132:1110.

31. Slaff and Brubaker. *The AIDS Epidemic* (New York: Warner Books, 1985), p. 40.

32. J. Weber, "Is AIDS an Epidemic Form of African Kaposi's Sarcoma?": Discussion Paper, *J Roy Soc Med* 1984;77:572-575.

33. J. Laurence, "The Immune System in AIDS", *Scientific American* 1985;253:90.

34. P. J. Buchanan and J. Gordon Muir, "Gay Times and Diseases", *The American Spectator,* vol. 17, no. 8, August 1984.

35. "Recommendations for Protection against Viral Hepatitis", *MMWR* 1985;34:pp.313-335.

36. Ostrow, op. cit., p. 117.

37. Kassler, *Gay Men's Health* (New York: Harper & Row, 1983), p. 38.

38. Ostrow, op. cit., p. 204.

39. Ma and Armstrong, op. cit., p. 100.

40. Kassler, op. cit., p. 39.

41. M. J. Alter and D. P. Francis, "Hepatitis B Virus Transmission between Homosexual Men: A Model for the Acquired Immunodeficiency Syndrome (AIDS)", in Ma and Armstrong, op. cit., pp. 97-106.

42. M. Seligman et al., "AIDS—An Immunologic Reevaluation", *N Eng J Med* 1984;311:1286-1291.

43. Jaffe et al., "National Case-Control Study: part 1"; p. 149 citing N. E. Reiner et al., "Asymptomatic Rectal Mucosal Lesions and Hepatitis B Surface Antigen at Sites of Sexual Contact in Homosexual Men with Persistent Hepatitis B Virus Infection: Evidence for de facto parenteral transmission", *Ann of Int Med* 1982; 96:170-173.

44. Ostrow, op. cit., p. 118, citing L. B. Self et al., "Hepatic Diseases in Asymptomatic Parenteral Narcotic Drug Abusers: A Veterans Administration Collaborative Study", *Am J Med Sci* 1975;270:41-47.

45. *Lancet,* 17 October, 1981.

46. K. M. De Cock et al., "Fulminant Delta Hepatitis in Chronic Hepatitis B Infection", *JAMA* 1984;252:2746-2748.

47. H. L. Kazal et al., "The Gay Bowel Syndrome. Clinico-pathologic Correlation in 260 Cases", *Ann Clin Lab Sci* 1976;6:184.

48. Buchanan and Muir, op. cit., p. 3.

49. Oscar Felsenfeld, *The Epidemiology of Tropical Diseases* (Ill.: Charles C. Thomas, 1966), pp. 395-397.

50. L. Corey and K. K. Holmes, "Sexual Transmission of Hepatitis A in Homosexual Men", *N Eng J Med* 1980;302:435-438.

51. Kassler, op. cit., p. 52.

52. A. Rompalo and H. Hunter Handsfield, "Overview of Sexually Transmitted Diseases in Homosexual Men", in Ma and Armstrong, op. cit., p. 8.

53. C. B. Panosian and S. L. Gorbach, "Bacterial Diarrhea in Homosexual Men", in Ma & Armstrong, op. cit., pp. 63-76.

54. H. W. Jaffe, "National Case-Control Study: Part 2", p. 145.

55. D. Williams, "Parasitic Infectious Diseases as Sexually Transmitted Infections", in Ma and Armstrong, op. cit., p. 78.

56. D. Abrams & R. Pearce, "AIDS and parasitism", *Lancet,* 23 June 1984, p. 1411.

57. Ma and Armstrong, op. cit., p. 6.

58. M. F. Rogers et al., "National Case-Control Study of Kaposi's Sarcoma and Pneumocystis Carinii Pneumonia in Homosexual Men: Part 2, Laboratory Results", *Ann of Int Med* 1983;99:151-158.

59. M. S. Gottlieb et al., "The Acquired Immunodeficiency Syndrome", *Ann of Int Med* 1983;99:208-220.

60. Ostrow, op. cit., p. 204.

61. Gottlieb, op. cit., p. 212.

62. Ibid., p. 209-210.

63. Ma and Armstrong, op. cit., p. 220.

64. Ibid., p. 7.

65. Ostrow, op. cit., p. 147.

66. Siegal and Siegal, *AIDS: The Medical Mystery* (New York: Grove Press, 1983), p. 2.

67. Ma and Armstrong, op. cit., p. 251.

68. Bobby Hilliard, "A 'Widow's' Story: Life after Your Lover Has Died of AIDS", *The Advocate,* 28 May 1985, p. 5.

69. Bell and Weinberg, op. cit., p. 312.

70. Ibid., p. 239.

71. *Time,* 21 October 1985.

72. J. Gross, "AIDS Epidemic Places Spotlight on Bathhouses", *New York Times,* 14 October 1985, p. 16.

73. Rueda, op. cit., p. 37.

74. Jaffe et al., "National Case-Control Study: part 1"; p. 146.

75. J. Gross, op. cit., p. 16.

76. L. McKusick et al., "AIDS and Sexual Behavior Reported by Gay Men in San Francisco", *Amer J of Pub Health* 1985;75:493-496.

77. "Update: Acquired Immunodeficiency Syndrome in the San Francisco Cohort Study, 1978-1985", *MMWR* 1985;34:573-575.

78. H. W. Jaffe et al., "The Acquired Immunodeficiency Syndrome in a Cohort of Homosexual Men", *Ann of Int Med* 1985; 103:210-214.

79. Slaff, op. cit., p. 184.

80. J. W. Curran, "The Epidemiology and Prevention of the Acquired Immunodeficiency Syndrome", *Ann of Int Med* 1985;103:657-662.

81. J. Sonnabend et al., "Acquired Immunodeficiency Syndrome, Opportunistic Infections, and Malignancies in Male Homosexuals: A Hypothesis of Etiologic Factors in Pathogenesis", *JAMA* 1983; 249:2370-2374.

Chapter 3

AIDS Spread into the General Population: The Time Bomb is Ticking

1. Siegal and Siegal, *AIDS: The Medical Mystery* (New York: Grove Press, 1983), p. 202.

2. Cory SerVaas, M.D., *The Saturday Evening Post,* January-February 1986, p. 107.

3. J. F. Grutsch and A. D. J. Robertson, "The Coming of AIDS", *The American Spectator,* March 1986, pp. 12-15.

4. A. Ellrodt et al., "Isolation of Human T-Lymphotropic Retrovirus (LAV) from Zairian Married Couple, One with AIDS, One with Prodromes", *Lancet,* 23 June 1984, pp. 1383-1385. R. W. Wykoff, "Female-to-Male Transmission of the AIDS Agent", *Lancet,* 2 November 1985, pp. 1017-1018.

5. N. Clumeck et al., "Seroepidemiological Studies of HTLV-III Antibody Prevalence among Selected Groups of Heterosexual Africans", *JAMA* 1985;254:2599-2602.

6. F. Brun-Vezinet, et al., "Prevalence of Antibodies to Lymphadenopathy-Associated Retrovirus in African Patients with AIDS", *Science* 1984;226:453-456.

7. J. Weber, "Is AIDS an Epidemic Form of Kaposi's Sarcoma?" *J Roy Soc Med* 1984;77:572-575.

8. *Discover,* December 1985, p. 52.

9. A. Ellrodt, op. cit., p. 1383.

10. *Discover,* December 1985, p. 52.

11. P. Van De Perre et al., "Acquired Immunodeficiency Syndrome in Rwanda", *Lancet,* 14 July 1984, pp. 62-65. P. Piot et al., "Acquired Immunodeficiency Syndrome in a Heterosexual Population in Zaire", *Lancet,* 14 July 1984, pp. 65-69.

12. P. Van De Perre et al., op. cit., p. 65.

13. P. Piot, op. cit., pp. 65-69.

14. P. Van De Perre, op. cit., p. 62, 65.

15. P. Piot, op. cit., p. 65.

16. Seale, "AIDS Virus Infection: Prognosis and Transmission", JAMA 1985;78:615.

17. K. M. De Cock, "AIDS: an old disease from Africa?" *British Med Journal* 1984;289:306-308.

18. Siegal and Siegal, op. cit., pp. 119-120.

19. A. C. Bayley et al., "HTLV-III Serology Distinguishes Atypical and Endemic Kaposi's Sarcoma In Africa", *Lancet,* 16 February 1985, pp. 359-361.

20. R. J. Biggar et al., "ELISA HTLV Retrovirus Antibody Reactivity Associated with Malaria and Immune Complexes in Healthy Africans", *Lancet,* 7 September 1985, pp. 520-523.

21. Slaff and Brubaker, *The AIDS Epidemic* (New York: Warner Books, 1985), p. 182.

22. D. J. Volsky et al., "Antibodies to HTLV-III/LAV in Venezuelan Patients with Acute Malarial Infections", *N Eng J Med* 1986; 314:647.

23. Seale, op. cit., pp. 614-615.

24. K. H. Mayer, "Medical Consequences of the Inhalation of Volatile Nitrites", in Ostrow et al., *Sexually Transmitted Diseases in Homosexual Men* (New York: Plenum Books, 1983), pp. 237-242.

25. H. W. Jaffe et al., "National Case-Control Study of Kaposi's Sarcoma and Pneumocystis Carinii Pneumonia in Homosexual Men: Part 1, Epidemiologic Results", *Ann of Int Med* 1983;99:145-146.

26. Siegal and Siegal, op. cit., p. 98.

27. J. R. Carlson et al., "AIDS Serology Testing in Low- and High-Risk Groups", *JAMA* 1985;253:3405-3408.

28. Slaff and Brubaker, op. cit., pp. 74-75.

29. L. B. Self et al., "Hepatic Diseases in Asymptomatic Parenteral Narcotic Drug Abusers: A Veterans Administration Collaborative Study." *Am J Med Sci* 1975;270:41-47 cited in Ostrow, op. cit., p. 135.

30. C. R. M. Hay et al., "Progressive Liver Disease in Haemophilia: An Understated Problem?" *Lancet,* 29 June 1985, pp. 1495-1498.

31. G. Ruggiero et al., "Liver Disease in Hemophiliacs: Etiological and Biochemical Data on 159 Cases from Our Geographical Area", *Hepato-gastroenterol* 1985;32:57-60.

32. Buchanan and Muir, "Gay Times and Diseases", *The American Spectator,* 8 (August 1984):3.

33. *Dallas Gay News,* 20 May 1983.

34. R. Yomtovian, "HTLV-III Antibody Testing: The False Negative Rate", *JAMA* 1986;255:609.

35. M. W. Ross et al., "Characteristics of homosexual Men Who Donate Blood", *Med J of Australia* 1985;142:343-344."

36. "The Battle against AIDS: Testing for HTLV-III", Lifetime Cable Network: 24 March 1985; 7:00–9:00 PM CST.

37. Slaff and Brubaker, op. cit., pp. 201; 251–252.

38. M. Chase, "Bad Blood", *Wall Street Journal,* 12 March 1984.

39. J. B. Schorr et al., "Prevalence of HTLV-III Antibody in American Blood Donors", *N Eng J Med* 1985;313:384–385.

40. "Blood Donors at High Risk of Transmitting the Acquired Immune Deficiency Syndrome", *Br Med J* 1985;290:749–750.

41. S. H. Landesman et al., "Special Report—The AIDS Epidemic", *N Eng J Med* 1985;312:521–525, citing B. L. Evatt et al., "Coincidental Appearance of LAV/HTLV-III Antibodies in Hemophiliacs and the Onset of the AIDS Epidemic", *N Eng J Med* 1985;312:483–486.

42. S. L. Sivak and G. P. Wormer, "How Common Is HTLV-III Infection in the United States?" *N Eng J Med* 1985;313:1352–1353.

43. C. Harris et al., "Immunodeficiency in Female Partners of Men with the Acquired Immunodeficiency Syndrome", *N Eng J Med* 1983;308:1181–1184. R. R. Redfield et al., "Frequent Transmission of HTLV-III among Spouses of Patients with the AIDS–Related Complex and AIDS", *JAMA* 1985;253:1571–1573.

44. J. C. Petricciani et al., "An Analysis of Serum Samples Positive for HTLV-III Antibodies", *N Eng J Med* 1985;313:47–48.

45. J. W. Curran, "The Epidemiology and Prevention of the Acquired Immunodeficiency Syndrome", *Ann of Int Med* 1985;103:659.

46. *Newsweek,* 12 August 1985, p. 22 (Source: Centers for Disease Control).

47. G. A. Ahronheim, "The Transmission of AIDS", *Nature* 1985;

313:534, citing G. M. Shearer and A. S. Rabson, *Nature* 1984; 308:230.

48. Slaff and Brubaker, op. cit., pp. 173-175.

49. J. Laurence, "The Immune System in AIDS", *Scientific American* 1985;253:90.

50. R. B. Pearce & D. I. Abrams, "AIDS and Parasitism", *Lancet,* 23 June 1985, p. 1411.

51. Advertisement by Merck Sharp & Dohme for the Hepatitis B vaccine, *N Eng J Med,* 20 January 1983, citing A. E. Denes et al., "Hepatitis B Infection in Physicians: Results of a Nationwide Serepidemiologic Survey", *JAMA* 1978;239:210-212.

52. R. T. Ravenholt, "Role of Hepatitis B Virus in Acquired Immunodeficiency Syndrome", *Lancet* 1983; ii:885-886.

53. P. Van De Perre et al., op. cit., p. 65.

54. J. Cohen et al., "Opportunistic AIDS", *Lancet* 1984;ii:1209-10.

55. Seale, op. cit., p. 614.

56. Grutsch and Robertson, op. cit., p. 13.

57. L. Montagnier, C. Dauget, C. Axlerblin et al., "New Type of Retrovirus Isolated from Patients Presenting with Lymphadenopathy or Acquired Immunodeficiency Syndrome: Structural and Antigenic Relatedness with Equine Infectious Anemia Virus", *Ann Virol* (Inst Pasteur) 1984;135(E):119-134.

58. "Heterosexual Transmission of Human T-Lymphotropic Virus Type III/Lymphadenopathy-Associated Virus", *MMWR* 1985;34: 561-563.

59. J. W. Curran, op. cit., p. 658.

60. C. Harris et al., op. cit., pp. 1181-1184.

61. R. R. Redfield et al., "Frequent Transmission of HTLV-III Among Spouses of Patients with AIDS–Related Complex and AIDS", *JAMA* 1985;253:1571-1573.

62. R. R. Redfield et al., "Heterosexually Acquired HTLV-III/LAV Disease (AIDS–Related Complex and AIDS) Epidemiologic Evidence for Female-to-Male Transmission", *JAMA* 1985;254:2094-2096, citing G. Papaevangelou et al., "Source of Infection Due to Hepatitis B Virus in Greece", *J Infect Dis* 1983;147:987-989.

63. "More Heterosexual Spread of HTLV-III Virus Seen", Editorial, *JAMA* 1985 253:3377-3379.

64. The *Advocate,* 29 October 1985, p. 22.

65. Slaff and Brubaker, op. cit., p. 6.

66. D. P. Francis et al., "The Natural History of Infection with the Lymphadenopathy-Associated Virus Human T-Lymphotropic Virus Type III", *Ann of Int Med* 1985;103:720.

67. G. J. Stewart et al., "Transmission of Human T-Cell Lymphotropic Virus Type III (HTLV-III) by Artificial Insemination by Donor", *Lancet,* 14 September 1985, pp. 581-584.

68. Buchanan and Muir, op. cit., p. 3.

69. *Moral Majority Report* (Washington, D.C.), February 1985, p. 16.

70. Slaff and Brubaker, op. cit., p. 61.

71. Tanne, "The Last Word on Avoiding AIDS", *New York Magazine,* 7 October 1985, p. 33.

72. S. I. Sivak et al., "How Common Is HTLV-III Infection in the United States?" *N Eng J Med* 1985;313:1352.

73. R. O. Hawkins, Jr. "Women Who Prefer Gay Men", *Medical Aspects of Human Sexuality,* July 1985, p. 192, citing A. E. Moses

and R. O. Hawkins, Jr., *Counseling Lesbian Women and Gay Men: A Life Issues Approach,* (St. Louis: CV Mosby, 1982).

74. Bell and Weinberg, *Homosexualities: A Study of Diversity among Men and Women* (New York: Simon and Schuster, 1978) p. 286, 162.

75. H. W. Jaffe et al., "National Case-Control Study of Kaposi's Sarcoma and Pneumocystis Carinii Pneumonia in Homosexual Men: part 1, Epidemiologic Results", *Ann Int Med* 1983;99:145-151.

76. W. Winkelstein et al., "Potential for Transmission of AIDS-Associated Retrovirus from Bisexual Men in San Francisco to Their Female Sexual Contacts", *JAMA* 1986;255:901.

77. W. A. Haseltine (response to a letter to the editor), *N Eng J Med* 1985;314:55-56.

Chapter 4
Casual Transmission—An Underrated Danger?

1. A. Fauci, "The Acquired Immune Deficiency Syndrome—The Ever-Broadening Clinical Spectrum", *JAMA* 1983;249:2375-2376.

2. "Precautions in the Handling of Clinical and Laboratory AIDS Materials", *MMWR* 1982;43:577-579.

3. *MMWR,* 15 November 1985, "Recommendations for Preventing Transmission of Infection with HTLV-III/LAV in the Workplace", pp. 682-695.

4. M. Stanton Evans, "AIDS Horror Story Worsens", *Human Events,* 30 November 1985, p. 7. "Summary: Recommendations for Preventing Transmission of Infection with HTLV-III/LAV in the Workplace, Leads from the *MMWR*", *JAMA* 1985;254:3023-3026.

5. William F. Buckley, Jr., *National Review,* 18 October 1985, p. 63.

6. *JAMA* 1985;254;21:3024.

7. *MMWR,* 7 June 1985, p. 323.

8. "The Acquired Immunodeficiency Syndrome, Commentary", The Council on Scientific Affairs, *JAMA* 1984;252:2037-2043.

9. T. Jonckheer et al., "Cluster of HTLV-III/LAV Infection in an African Family", *Lancet* 16 February 1985, pp. 400-401.

10. "Fighting a Scourge", *Wall Street Journal,* 5 August 1985.

11. "Medical News", *JAMA* 22/29 November 1985, p. 2867.

12. J. M. Jason et al., "HTLV-III/LAV Antibody and Immune Status of Household Contacts and Sexual Partners of Persons with Hemophilia", *JAMA,* 10 January 1986, pp. 212-215.

13. P. J. Grob et al., *Lancet,* 28 November 1981, pp. 1218-1220.

14. *MMWR,* 8 February 1985, pp. 73, 74.

15. L. A. Lettau et al., *JAMA,* 21 February 1986, pp. 934-937.

16. Slaff and Brubaker, *The AIDS Epidemic* (New York: Warner Books, 1985), p. 236.

17. G. T. Werner et al., "Prevalence of Serological Hepatitis A and B Markers in a Rural Area of Northern Zaire", *Am J Trop Med Hyg* 1985;34;3:620-624.

18. M. J. Blaser, *JAMA,* 1986;255:463, 464.

19. J. F. Grutsch and A. D. J. Robertson, "The Coming of AIDS", *American Spectator,* March 1986, p. 13.

20. J. E. Groopman et al., "HTLV-III in Saliva of People with AIDS-Related Complex and Healthy Homosexual Men at Risk for AIDS", *Science,* 24 October 1984, pp. 447-449.

21. CDC, 11 January 1985.

22. S. Z. Salahuddin et al., "HTLV-III in symptom-free seronegative persons", *Lancet* 1984;ii:1418.

23. *Washington Post,* 8 September 1985.

24. T. Tervo et al., "Recovery of HTLV-III from Contact Lenses", *Lancet,* 15 February 1986, pp. 379, 380. Eye care professionals desiring further information are referred to the article by Dr. Robert Gallo and other researchers, "Human T-cell Leukemia/Lymphotropic Virus Type III in the Conjunctival Epithelium of a Patient with AIDS", *American Journal of Ophthalmology,* 100, 1985, pp. 507-509.

25. Slaff and Brubaker, op. cit., p. 42.

26. F. Barre-Sinoussi et al., "Resistance of AIDS Virus at Room Temperature", *Lancet,* 28 September 1985, pp. 721-722.

27. *JAMA* Medical News, 22/29 November 1985, p. 2866.

28. L. Resnick et al., "Stability and Inactivation of HTLV-III/LAV under Clinical and Laboratory Experiments", *JAMA* 1985;225: 1887-1891.

29. Siegal and Siegal, *AIDS: The Medical Mystery,* p. 97.

30. K. M. Cahill, *The AIDS Epidemic* (New York: St. Martin's Press, 1983), pp. 126, 135.

31. G. M. Shearer, "Other Factors to Consider in Infantile AIDS", *N Eng J Med* 1984;311:189-190.

32. *MMWR,* 6 December 1985.

33. *Sexually Transmitted Diseases:* 1980 *Status Report,* NIAID Study Group, U.S. Department of Health and Human Services, Public Health Service, National Institutes of Health NIH Publication No. 81-2213, p. 136.

34. E. Gonczol et al., "Cytomegalovirus Replicates in Differentiated but Not in Undifferentiated Human Embryonal Carcinoma Cells", *Science* 1984;224:159-161, citing S. Stagno et al., *Semin. Perinatol.* 7, 31 (1983).

35. Kassler, *Gay Men's Health* (New York: Harper and Row, 1983), p. 21.

36. Y. M. Felman et al., "Kaposi's Sarcoma and Other Rare Malignancies in Homosexual Men", citing W. L. Drew et al., "Prevalence of Cytomegalovirus in Homosexual Men", *J Infect Dis* 1981; 143:188, in Ostrow, Sandholzer and Felman, *Sexually Transmitted Diseases in Homosexual Men* (New York: Plenum, 1983), pp. 197-212.

37. "Update: Treatment of Cryptosporidiosis in Patients with Acquired Immunodeficiency Syndrome (AIDS)", *MMWR,* 9 March 1984, pp. 117-119.

38. B. S. Gingold, "Gay Bowel Syndrome—An Overview", in Ma and Armstrong, *The Acquired Immune Deficiency Syndrome and Infections of Homosexual Men* (New York; Yorke Medical Books, 1984), p. 60.

39. Ostrow, op. cit., p. 208.

40. Ma and Armstrong, op. cit., p. 78.

41. P. Van De Perre et al., "Antibody to HTLV-III in Blood Donors in Central Africa", *Lancet,* 9 February 1985, pp. 336-337; cf., R. C. Brunham et al., "Depression of the Lymphocytes Transformation Response to Microbial Antigens and to Phytohemagglutinin during Pregnancy", *J Clin Invest* 1983;72:1629-38.

42. "Recommendations for Assisting in the Prevention of Perinatal Transmission of HTLV-III/LAV and Acquired Immunodeficiency Syndrome", *MMWR,* 6 December 1985.

43. Slaff and Brubaker, op. cit., p. 185.

44. P. A. Palsson, *Slow Virus Diseases of Animals and Man,* edited by R. H. Kimberlin, (Amsterdam: North Holland Publishing Co., 1976), p. 37.

45. M. J. Blaset, *JAMA,* 1986; 255:463, 464.

46. David A. Noebel et al., *Special Report: AIDS* (Manitou Springs, Col.: Summit Press, 1986), p. 126.

47. J.-M. Ziza et al., "Lymphadenopathy-Associated Virus Isolated from Bronchoalveolar Lavage Fluid in AIDS-Related Complex with Lymphoid Interstitial Pneumonitis", *N Eng J Med* 1985;313:183.

48. *J Roy Soc Med,* February 1986, p. 122.

49. *Wall Street Journal,* 13 March 1986.

50. Cedric A. Nims, *The Pathogenesis of Infectious Disease* (New York: Academic Press, 1977), pp. 27-28.

51. Richard Restak, "Worry about Survival of Society First; Then AIDS Victims' Rights", *Washington Post,* 8 September 1985.

Chapter 5
Fading Prospects for a Cure or Vaccine

1. A. G. Goodman et al., *The Pharmacological Basis of Therapeutics* (New York: Macmillan, 1980), p. 1240.

2. M. Seligman et al., "AIDS—An Immunologic Reevaluation", *N Eng J Med* 1984;311:1286-1292.

3. R. C. Gallo and F. Wong-Staal, "A Human T-Lymphotropic Retrovirus (HTLV-III) as the Cause of the Acquired Immunodeficiency Syndrome", *Ann of Int Med* 1985;103:679.

4. H. C. Lane and A. Fauci, "Immunologic Reconstitution in the

Acquired Immunodeficiency Syndrome", *Ann of Int Med* 1985;
103:714-718.

5. M. Essex et al., "Antigens of Human T-Lymphotropic Virus
Type III/Lymphadenopathy-Associated Virus", *Ann of Int Med* 1985;
103:700-703.

6. *JAMA,* 22/29 November 1985.

7. "AIDS-Associated Virus Yields Data to Intensifying Scientific
Study", *JAMA,* 22/29 November 1985, pp. 2865-2866.

8. Seale, "AIDS Virus Infection: Prognosis and Transmission",
JRSM 1985;78:614.

Chapter 6
The Specter of Continued AIDS Spread

1. S. L. Sivak and G. P. Wormer, "How Common Is HTLV-III
Infection in the United States", *N Eng J Med* 1985;313:1352-1353.

2. Hardy et al., "The Economic Impact of the First 10,000 Cases
nal of Acquired Immunodeficiency Syndrome in the United States",
JAMA 1986; 255:209-211.

3. *World Almanac Book of Facts, 1986* (New York: United Media
Enterprises, 1986), p. 333.

4. "Neurological Complications appear Often in AIDS", *JAMA*
1985:253:3379-3383.

5. C. V. Reyes, "Primary Malignant Lymphoma of the Brain in
Acquired Immune Deficiency Syndrome", *Acta Cytologica: The
Journal of Clinical Cytology and Cytopathology* 1985;29:85-86.
G. M. Shaw et al., "HTLV-III Infection in Brains of Children and
Adults with AIDS Encephalopathy", *Science* 1985;227:177-182.

6. "AIDS: A Growing Threat", *Time,* 12 August 1985, p. 47.

7. Hardy et al., op. cit, pp. 209-211.

8. "Acquired Immunodeficiency Syndrome," *Ann of Int Med* 1986; 104:575-581.

9. World Almanac, 1986, p. 788.

10. "Acquired Immunodeficiency Syndrome", *Ann of Int Med* 1986; 104:575-581.

11. *JAMA* 1984;252:2042.

12. Hardy, *op. cit.*, pp. 209-211.

13. Slaff and Brubaker, op. cit., pp. 162-163.

Chapter 7

The Major Obstacle to Halting AIDS Spread:
"Acquired Integrity Deficiency Syndrome"

1. Restak, "Worry about Survival of Society First; Then AIDS Victims' Rights", *Washington Post*, 8 September 1985.

2. Ibid.

3. D. Noebel et al., citing Dr. Olav H. Alvig, *American Medical News*, 20 December 1985.

4. See *JAMA*, 4 April 1986.

5. S. K. Dritz, "Medical Aspects of Homosexuality", *N Eng J Med* 1980;302:463-464.

6. J. C. Fletcher, "Artificial Insemination in a Lesbian: Ethical Considerations", *Arch Int Med* 1985;145:419-420.

7. Slaff and Brubaker, *The AIDS Epidemic* (New York: Warner, 1985), pp. 94-108.

8. "The Acquired Immunodeficiency Syndrome, Commentary, Council on Scientific Affairs", *JAMA* 1984;252:2042.

9. D. Noebel et al., *Special Report: AIDS* (Manitou Springs, Col.: Summit Press, 1986), pp. 109-111, taken from official testimony of Candice Comstive, R.N., before the Houston City Council, September 25, 1985.

10. *U.S. News and World Report,* 23 September 1985, p. 10.

11. Onofre, 434 N.Y.S.2d at 951. cited in Charles Rice, *Legalizing Homosexual Conduct: The Role of the Supreme Court in the Gay Rights Movement* (Cumberland, Va.: Center for Judicial Studies, 1984), pp. 19-20.

12. S. K. Dritz, op. cit., p. 464.

13. *New York Times,* 22 December 1985, p. 29.

14. T. B. Stoddard et al., *The Rights of Gay People* (New York: Bantam Books, 1983), p. 171.

15. "Court Says No Religion in the Marketplace", *Fundamentalist Journal,* November 1985, p. 69.

16. Rice, op. cit., pp. 2, 21.

17. Noebel et al., *Special Report: AIDS,* p. 18.

18. Ibid., pp. 16-17 citing *National Review,* 1 November 1985, p. 18.

19. Marlin Maddoux, *America Betrayed!* (Shreveport, La.: Huntington House, 1984), p. 93.

20. "Infection-Control Guidelines for Patients with the Acquired Immunodeficiency Syndrome (AIDS)", *N Eng J Med* 1983;309: 740-744.

21. *N Eng J Med,* 3 May 1984, p. 1194.

22. *Ibid.*

23. *Nature,* 26 October 1984, pp. 447-448.

24. National Coalition of Gay STD Services Fact Sheet, Arlington, Va., n.d., cited in Rueda, *The Homosexual Network,* p. 168.

25. Official Newsletter of the National Coalition of Gay STD Services 2 [Arlington, Va.: National Coalition of Gay STD Services, October 1980]:6, cited by Rueda, *The Homosexual Network,* p. 168.

26. Enrique Rueda, *The Homosexual Network: Private Lives and Public Policy* (Old Greenwich, Con.: Devin Adair, 1982), p. 168.

27. Ibid., p. 216.

28. For further examples of similar types of psychological coercion being used in classrooms throughout the United States see Phyllis Schlafly, ed., *Child Abuse in the Classroom* (Westchester, Ill.: Crossway Books, 1985).

29. Laud Humphreys, *Out of the Closets: The Sociology of Homosexual Liberation* (Englewood Cliffs, N.J.: Prentice-Hall, 1972), pp. 165-167.

30. Rueda, op. cit., p. 198.

31. Slaff and Brubaker, op. cit., p. 184.

32. "Recommendations for Protection against Viral Hepatitis", *MMWR,* 7 June 1985, pp. 322-323.

33. *New York Times,* 27 September 1985.

Chapter 8
Stopping the AIDS Juggernaut

1. J. H. Powell, Bring out Your Dead, *The Great Plague of Yellow Fever in Philadelphia in* 1793 (*Philadelphia: University of Pennsylvania Press,* 1949), p. 45.

2. *Freedom Report,* vol. 5, no. 1, January 1986, p. 5.

3. G. Muir, "AIDS: The Imperative for Discipline", *Texas Business,* December 1985, p. 16.

4. J. C. Beldekas, "Can AIDS Be Stopped?" *New York Native,* October 21-27, 1985, p. 21.

5. *New York Magazine,* 7 October 1985, p. 33.

6. Slaff and Brubaker, *The AIDS Epidemic* (New York: Warner, 1985), p. 245.

7. Rice, *Legalizing Homosexual Conduct* (Cumberland, Va.: Center for Judicial Studies, 1984), p. v.

8. Restak, "Worry about Survival of Society First; Then AIDS Victims' Rights", *Washington Post,* 8 September 1985.

9. *United States Code Service,* 42 USCS, The Public Health and Welfare (San Francisco: Bancroft-Whitney, 1978), Section 264, p. 363.

10. *Lancet,* 30 March 1985, p. 768.

11. R. Roemer and G. A. McKray, *Legal Aspects of Public Health* (New York: Greenwood Press, 1980), p. 10.

12. Siegal and Siegal, *AIDS: The Medical Mystery,* p. 146.

13. *Lancet,* 6 July 1985, p. 52.

14. *Discover,* December 1985, p. 53.

EPILOGUE
The Need for Sober Compassion

1. Dietrich Bonhoeffer, *Ethics* (New York: Macmillan, 1976), pp. 73-74.

2. J. C. Fletcher, "Artificial Insemination in a Lesbian: Ethical Considerations", *Arch Int Med* 1985;145:419-420.

3. Slaff and Brubaker, *The AIDS Epidemic* (New York: Warner Books, 1985), p. 213.

4. *Life,* July 1985, p. 19.

5. *Essays on Love* (Downers Grove, Ill.: Intervarsity Press, 1978), p. 35.

6. Carl Rowan, *Washington Post,* 28 May 1985.

7. *Fort Worth Star-Telegram,* 28 January 1986.

8. Fulton J. Sheen, *Treasure in Clay: The Autobiography of Fulton J. Sheen* (New York: Doubleday, 1980; available from Ignatius Press, San Francisco), pp. 203-204.

9. David R. Mace, "Is Chastity Outmoded?" *Woman's Home Companion,* September 1949, pp. 37-38, 101, cited in Evelyn Mills Duvall, *Why Wait Till Marriage* (New York: Association Press, 1970), pp. 92-93.

10. See Lev 18; Rom 1; I Cor 6, etc.

11. J. L. Fletcher, "Homosexuality: Kick and Kickback", *South Med J* 1984;77:149-150.

APPENDIX

1. Centers for Disease Control, Atlanta. "Revision of case definitions of AIDS for national reporting—United States", *MMWR* 1985; 34:373-375.

2. F. Barre-Sinoussi, M. T. Nugeyre, J. C. Chermann, "Resistance of AIDS virus at room temperature". *Lancet* 1985;ii:721-722.

AIDS UPDATE: 1987 Supplement

A world-wide AIDS epidemic will become so serious it will dwarf such earlier medical disasters as the Black Plague, smallpox and typhoid. If we can't make progress, we face the dreadful prospect of a world-wide death toll in the tens of millions a decade from now [emphasis added].

— Dr. Otis Bowen, Secretary of Health and Human Services[1]

Crisis Growing Worse

In this book every effort has been made intentionally to modify and understate the nature of the problem. The objection has been raised by some that the true severity of and potential for this disaster has been unnecessarily mollified. By others that unnecessary fears may be raised. Unfortunately, all forthcoming data indicate that the epidemic is even worse than has been reported. Dr. Halfdan Mahler, Director of the World Health Organization based in the United Nations states: "We're running scared." He said he could "not imagine a worse health problem in this century."

"We stand nakedly in front of a very serious pandemic as mortal as there has ever been", he continued. "I don't know of any greater killer than AIDS, not to speak of its psychological, social and economic maiming. . . . *Everything is getting worse and worse in AIDS and all of us have been underestimating it.*"

He said a year ago, at a news conference in Zambia, that people should keep AIDS in perspective relative to other diseases. Today he acknowledged that he had not had "a feeling for what was brewing with regard to AIDS".

"I thought wait and see—maybe its not as hot as some are making it appear", he said. "I definitely admit to a gross under-estimate." Dr. Mahler said that as many as *100 million people could be infected with the AIDS virus in five years.*[2]

In chapter six of this book it is contended that the implosion of the nation's health care system appears imminent. This concern is being borne out by experience. In the March 1987 issue of *Vanity Fair*, Dr. William Grace, chief of oncology at St. Vincent's Hospital in New York reports:

> Every ten to twelve months the number of AIDS patients doubles—everywhere. Right now at St. Vincent's, 45 medical beds—of our 316 beds available—are occupied by AIDS patients, and most of these are middle-class patients, not the drug users or others without medical coverage, who get sent to Bellevue. What happens next year, when we have ninety patients? And 180 the year after that? In four years we will have exhausted all the medical beds in New York.

Dr. Grace is absolutely blunt about it:

> *I think AIDS is going to devastate the American medical system.* Last year, coronary-bypass surgery cost $1 billion in this country—and that was very expensive. In 1985, the 12,000 patients with AIDS cost this country $6 billion. Do you realize that in five years there are going to be over a quarter of a million cases? The virus is already incubating in one million people, and what we're seeing now is that the incubation period can be eight or nine years. *We're also seeing that a steadily growing number of those with the virus are actually getting AIDS. We're also seeing other viruses like the AIDS virus—viruses that aren't even talked about in the press. There will be many, many more.* [3]

Disease Breaking out
of Previous Risk Groups

As delineated in Chapter 2 and elsewhere, AIDS is a disease that in the West has been primarily fostered and spread by male homosexuals/bisexuals. Barring effective health measures, the potential for massive spread from this group throughout the rest of the population does exist. A recent report in the Journal of the American Medical Association states: "There has been an increasing number of persons with AIDS whose only risk factor has been heterosexual contact with a person known to have AIDS or a person at risk for AIDS." [4] The anatomy of the female genitalia is apparently less predisposed to AIDS transmission than the fecal excretory tract.[5] It is clear, however, that normal heterosexual coitus, even if less efficient than sodomy, permits disease transmission.

A recent report by the CDC indicates that heterosexual transmission of AIDS is on the rise.[6] The number of infected women is rising as is the number of heterosexual males. A recent study of prostitutes in Washington D.C. indicates that 50% of them are active carriers of the AIDS virus. Evidence from Africa indicates that infected female prostitutes are conveying the disease to their partners. As reported in the Foreword of this book, Dr. William Haseltine of Harvard estimates that 20% to 30% of the college women in various areas of the United States are likely to contract the disease. Based on current epidemiological data, experts are now predicting that 25% of the population of Africa will be dead from AIDS within a little more than a decade.[7]

There is reason to believe, based on the existing trends of other sexually transmitted diseases, that AIDS may reach close to that proportion in the United States and other Western countries as well. The Public Health Service asserts that there will be 270,000 Americans dead or dying of AIDS by 1991 and that this figure underestimates the problem by at least 20% (54,000 persons) due to underreporting.

By 1995, the toll of dead and dying will have risen into the millions. Abstinence before marriage and fidelity afterwards are not completely reliable as the number of bisexual men infected with the virus is large and growing.

The Atlantic Monthly reports that: "Bisexuals have always been the big problem in tracing sexually transmitted diseases, according to Rick Reich, who spent several years working as a venereal disease case investigator in Los Angeles. 'In my experience,' he says, 'a certain kind of bisexual man is not immoral but amoral as regards sexual candor'."[8] Many bisexual men will not admit to their female partner(s) that they also have been involved in homosexuality and are at risk of transmitting AIDS. This along with the risk to males from infected women is one of the reasons why many people have been calling for a pre-marital AIDS blood test as has been done with syphilis.

Political Pressure Blocking
Effective Public Health Measures

It must be stressed that persons infected with the AIDS virus who as yet display no visible symptoms are infectious, i.e., able to transmit the disease. The CDC reports that infectious AIDS virus has been found "in blood, semen, saliva, tears, urine, cerebro-spinal fluid, brain tissue, and cervical secretions and is likely to be found in other fluids, secretions and tissues. . . . Direct contact of cuts, scratches, abrasions, or mucosal surfaces [eye, nose, mouth] with suspensions of virus or specimens containing live virus are considered potential routes of infection."[9] The risk of medical and nursing personnel acquiring AIDS infection through contact with an undiagnosed AIDS carrier who is a patient has therefore been a source of deep concern for those involved in primary patient care. A physician in *The British Medical Journal* cites a case in point:

> The time has come when we must ask people who are positive for HIV* antibody [infected with the AIDS virus] to carry an identity card in case they are injured and unable to warn anyone of their [infectious] antibody state.
>
> Recently a young man received a head injury and bled profusely. His parents tried to stop the bleeding and their hands were covered with his blood. The ambulanceman dressed his wound and took him with his parents to the emergency room. As the patient was constantly moving his head the nurse who was removing the bandage pricked her finger while unlocking the safety pin. The wound started to bleed again, and when his parents left the room the patient asked the medical and nursing staff to take extra precautions as he was positive for HIV antibody. . . .
>
> Even at this stage the patient insisted that his parents should not be told—a wish that had to be honored under the present rule of confidentiality. Accordingly, the parents were told that their son had an infection [of some kind, but not specifically AIDS]. . . .
>
> This episode raises various questions: 1) Why did the patient not warn his parents, the ambulanceman, or the hospital medical and

* HIV or Human Immunodeficiency Virus is now the commonly used term for the AIDS virus.

nursing staff of his infection immediately? 2) What could have been the effects had he been unconscious, undergone an operation and been placed in a hospital ward? 3) How much mental torture has been caused to the nursing staff, ambulance crew, and their families? 4) Should the families of people who are positive for HIV antibody be told?

I discussed the possibility of an identity card system with this patient. He agreed that it was a good idea and said that he would have no objection to carrying such a card.[10]

Apart from caring for patients with traumatic injuries such as the case above, medical personnel caring for patients with all types of illness may be exposed to blood, urine, feces and other potentially infective bodily fluids and secretions. Protecting the safety of medical personnel is one of the reasons that some medical professionals raised the idea of screening all patients for AIDS virus infection upon admission to hospitals.

Screening patients upon intake, and other issues such as instituting a pre-marital AIDS blood test and tracing the sexual contacts of infectious carriers were addressed at a conference in Atlanta, Georgia held in February of 1987.

At least, an *attempt* was made to address them. Homosexual militants disrupted meetings on several occasions. CDC director James Mason described the conference goal: "We're here to defeat a common enemy." But that goal, according to the *Medical World News*, seemed elusive.

The Lavender Hill Mob, a militant New York homosexual rights group tauntingly accused the CDC of "fascist tactics" and of placing too much emphasis on testing. A group shouting "silent no more!" broke up a meeting as Dr. Walter Dowdle, acting director of the CDC, attempted to deliver his closing remarks.

Testing and counseling is intended, as with all sexually transmitted diseases, to prevent further spread of the disease by increasing the number of known "contact points", asserted Dr. Ward Cates, Jr., CDC director of sexually transmitted diseases. In his prepared remarks, Dr. Cates noted that the vast majority of those infected are not yet aware that they are infectious carriers of the virus. "How do you reach them? To me that's what this conference has been all about.'' (''Mandatory AIDS Testing Fizzles at Raucous CDC Conference . . . '', *Medical World News*, 20 March 1987.)

The New York Times reported, however, that

> concern over the need to protect people who are infected with the AIDS virus from loss of jobs, housing, insurance and the right to enter public places was a dominant theme on the opening day of the conference.[11]

By conference end, all suggestions regarding the testing of hospital patients, pre-marital blood tests or contact tracing were drowned out by a vociferous chorus emphasizing the civil liberties of AIDS carriers.

AIDS Dementia: Implications for Public Policy

As covered in the analysis, *A Critical Evaluation of the Surgeon General's Report on AIDS*,* the ability of the AIDS virus to devastate the brain apart from immune deficiency is increasingly being recognized. The CDC now acknowledges AIDS-virus dementia as a manifestation of AIDS related complex (ARC).[12] (Persons dying as a result of AIDS dementia without severe immune suppression are still not reported as having AIDS.)

As the reader may recall from Chapter 2, AIDS virus attack of the brain causes loss of short term memory, mental confusion, loss of muscular coordination, mutism, personality disintegration, coma and finally death. It can and does occur apart from impairment of the immune system. A NOVA documentary on AIDS aired on PBS gives a first hand insight into one of the effects of AIDS dementia:

> Narrator: The AIDS virus doesn't just attack the immune system. Scientists now know it can also infect the brain.

* See order form in back of the book.

Dr. Robert Gallo: Infecting the brain, it can cause dementia and it can cause death, directly. These are cases that often go unreported, because they're not showing up as AIDS, but as brain disease. People don't often know the virus is there. . . .

Narrator: Some people infected with the virus can experience mental problems long before they show serious symptoms of disease. This volunteer, for example, has only a mildly damaged immune system.

Man: I used to have a real good memory. You could give me a list of a hundred like items in a store and I could read'em back to you frontward, backward, what sequence they were in, all that stuff, you know, and uh, I mean now it's like, I go to the store for five items and I forget three of them, you know.

Narrator: Brain scans reveal the damage that can be done by the virus. The brain literally shrinks and fluid, shown here in black, fills the space. Over 50% of AIDS patients may ultimately suffer from dementia.

Dr. Alexandra Beckett, Massachusetts General Hospital: The complaints that we've most often heard are that people are having difficulty concentrating. We have commonly had people describe episodes during which they have sudden strong emotion, unpre-cipitated by anything they can point to. And that they feel *they are performing less well than they used to at tasks that they are quite familiar with.*

Narrator: And the indications are that brain damage *is* something many people infected with the AIDS virus will increasingly have to face.[13]

Dr. Paul Volberding, head of AIDS services at San Francisco General Hospital asserts:

It is entirely reasonable to speculate that *everyone* who is sero-positive [infected with the virus] will develop central nervous system complications. We are seeing an increasing number of signs of this on our ward. They take the form of varying degrees of dementia [emphasis added].[14]

Various other neurological complications have been associated with AIDS virus infection.[15] Recently a case was reported in which a twenty-nine year old homosexual male infected with the AIDS virus developed acute myelopathy:

On the fifth day after admission to the hospital he reported that his right leg felt stiff, and his gait became increasingly unsteady. . . . Later the same day he suffered an episode of generalized shaking of the legs and experienced difficulty in voiding urine. He seemed mentally slow. . . .

Over the next two weeks he continued to experience spasms of uncontrolled shaking of the legs. In addition, he described severe lancinating pains in his back which he likened to electric shocks. . . . Blood and cerebrospinal fluid were cultured, and the AIDS virus was isolated from both sources. . . . Although the primary site of damage was the spinal cord, there were subtle signs of dysfunction at a higher level (impaired mental activity).[16]

The medical establishment has been outspoken in its insistence that AIDS virus carriers, ARC and AIDS patients should not be excluded from any form of employment based on the danger of contagion. Homosexual groups are using AIDS as a pretext to force states which do not have anti-discrimination statutes to ban discrimination in hiring based on the real or perceived risk of an individual's being an infectious AIDS carrier. They are attempting to get the courts to ban discrimination based on protection of such individuals as being "handicapped". Attorney Jeffrey Madoff underscores how this type of ruling may be applied:

Even in jurisdictions where the statute only addresses protection of "disabled" individuals, and does not extend to protecting persons "regarded" or "perceived" as being handicapped, a cause of action may arise on behalf of persons *merely perceived to be members of risk groups* (e.g., homosexuals, drug abusers, Haitians), on the ground that the employer's action against such individuals is motivated by the same *unlawful prejudice* as would be the case if the individual was an actual AIDS sufferer [emphasis added].[17]

In spite of the present attempts to ban discrimination in employment based on AIDS carriers being given "handicap" status, it is clear that the destructive effect of the AIDS virus on the brain can and will have an adverse effect on job performance. Madoff continues:

In virtually every jurisdiction with a handicap discrimination statute, discrimination in employment decisions against the disabled is lawful if the physical requirements of the job cannot be performed by the individual at the time the individual is being evaluated for employment or his performance is being reviewed.[18]

It is essential that the reality of impaired job performance be brought under careful scrutiny when determining the suitability of infected employees or job applicants for various occupations. A pilot, surgeon or nurse who is slowly, almost imperceptibly suffering neurological damage from the effects of the AIDS virus on the brain poses a real danger to the lives of others. The threat to public safety posed by such individuals raises some critical questions which need to be addressed posthaste.

Should an airline company wait until a pilot causes a fatal accident while suffering momentary mental confusion before deciding he is no longer fit for the job? Should a hospital wait until a surgeon accidentally kills his patient due to impaired mental acuity before determining he had better lay down his scalpel? Should an infected nurse only be restricted *after* he or she forgetfully gives patients the wrong and possibly fatal medication?

An AIDS infected locomotive engineer or school bus driver who suddenly "forgets" which signal switch or sign means what is also an alarming prospect. Some time ago, there was a major train accident in the Northeastern United States involving a number of fatalities and scores of injured persons. Drug usage by the crew was cited as a significant element in the tragedy. This has evoked strong demands for blood testing of employees to ensure against such tragedies in the future.

At the very least, it would seem highly appropriate for those in occupations where mental impairment would endanger the lives of others to be periodically screened for AIDS virus infection. Tests for mental acuity and muscle coordination ought to be given to those infected to determine suitability for performing occupational tasks. Those who have developed mental impairment due to AIDS virus infection of the brain could perhaps be given jobs where their "handicap" would not endanger the lives of others.

For that matter, the prospect of an individual driving a motor vehicle while in a demented AIDS induced stupor is also a source of deep concern. Should society wait until fatalities mount from

AIDS brain impaired drivers before taking steps to prevent such carnage?

However the above situations may be handled, the neurological impairment induced by the AIDS virus is certain to intensify the controversy involving AIDS carriers in the workplace.*

The Potential for Casual Spread of AIDS

When Professor William Haseltine of the Harvard Medical School recently gave his university audience some of the scientific facts about AIDS, there was a stunned silence. Anyone "who tells you categorically that AIDS is not contracted by saliva is not telling you the truth. AIDS may in fact be transmissible by tears, saliva, bodily fluids, and mosquito bites. There are sure to be cases", he continued, "of proved transmission through casual contact."[19]

Up to the present time, most studies would indicate that medical workers and family members having close non-sexual contact with body fluids and secretions of AIDS infected patients and relatives are not at unusually high risk of acquiring AIDS virus infection. There are a number of cases cited in medical literature, however, which emphasize the need for caution when coming into contact with potentially infective tissues, fluids, secretions and insects. The British Medical Journal *Lancet* presented the case in which

a 24-year old student nurse pricked the fleshy part of her index finger with a needle used to take blood from an AIDS patient. *No injection of blood was noted at the time* (July 12, 1985). She was HIV antibody negative 1 month later. On September 8th she presented with fever, a macular eruption affecting progressively her face, arms and thorax. . . . She had lymphopenia and thrombocytopenia. An

* "Preliminary studies from several groups showed up to a 30% incidence of early abnormalities of cognitive function in *apparently healthy HIV-seropositive homosexual men.* . . . More worrying was the high prevalence of abnormalities in the cerebrospinal fluid: in patients with AIDS-related complex about one-half have evidence of the intracerebral synthesis of antibodies specific for the AIDS virus . . . " [emphasis added]. "Conference Report: Second International Conference on AIDS", *The Medical Journal of Australia*, 1986; 145:524-529.

AIDS blood test at that time was negative. She was HIV seropositive in January, 1986. . . .

The woman's husband was tested in January and April, 1986, and was negative. This young woman has not had repeated transfusions, is not an intravenous drug user, and has not had extramarital sexual relations.

The infectious episode of September, 1985, can probably be attributed to an acute HIV infection. The 2-month incubation period may be explained by *the small quantity of virus* introduced; *there was merely a puncture wound without injection of contaminated blood.*[20]

The New England Journal of Medicine has also reported a well-documented case of AIDS virus infection occurring in a health care worker after a needlestick injury.[21]

A case involving transmission of AIDS virus infection between two brothers through a bite has also been reported. A little boy contracted AIDS from a contaminated blood transfusion found to have been donated by a homosexual. Shortly after the child's death from AIDS, his brother, three years older, was found to have become infected with the virus. The physicians presenting the report state:

One possible route of virus transmission was a bite on the older brother's forearm by the younger child about six months before he died. The mother had seen teeth imprints on the skin but no bleeding or haematoma. This observation suggests that even minor bites by HIV infected children may carry the risk of virus transmission. Parents, teachers, and other people responsible for HIV-infected children should be aware of this possibility and try to prevent spread of the virus by this route.[22]

Survival of HIV in the Common Bedbug

The potential for insect spread of AIDS lentivirus infection in humans is consonant with the transmission of the lentivirus causing equine infectious anemia in horses.

Equine infectious anemia virus [EIAV] is effectively transmitted
in a mechanical fashion by blood-feeding insects, especially horse-
flies. . . .
    Understanding the mechanical transmission of EIAV by blood-
feeding insects may be of extreme importance *when* AIDS viruses
are documented to be vector transmitted.[23]

Now a study from *The Lancet* has presented evidence that
mechanical transmission of HIV can occur between humans, especially young children, via bedbugs. "The survival of HIV for
one hour in the common bedbug (*C Lectularius*) following the
feed on a blood virus mixture suggests that mechanical transmission of the virus between human beings could be carried out by
bedbugs."[24]

AIDS Virus Infection of Lung Tissue

As cited on pages 118-120 of this book, the lentivirus which causes
degenerative brain and lung disease (maedi-visna) in sheep is
spread by coughing while the animals are in close contact. A case
was also described in which the AIDS virus was found in the lung
washings (bronchoalveolar lavage fluid) of a patient with AIDS-
related complex who had a resultant inflammation of the interstitial
tissues of the lungs. The question is raised as to whether inhaling
quantities of the AIDS virus could result in a dangerous inflammation of lung tissue (Chronic Lymphoid Interstitial Pneumonitis
or CLIP). A study in the March 1987 *American Journal of
Medicine* describes two cases of lymphocytic interstitial pneumonitis in association with infection by AIDS-related complex. The
researchers found that:

> The ratio of the concentrations of HTLV-III/LAV-specific IgG to
> total IgG in the bronchoalveolar lavage fluid *was higher than that of
> the peripheral blood.* . . .
>   These findings confirm a previous preliminary report describing
> HTLV-III/LAV antigen and antibody in bronchoalveolar lavage
> fluid from a patient with lymphocytic interstitial pneumonitis and
> AIDS-related complex and are consistent with the hypothesis that

lymphocytic interstitial pneumonitis *is sometimes associated with AIDS virus infection of pulmonary tissue that evokes a specific humoral response locally in the lung.* . . .

HTLV-III/LAV is morphologically and genetically related to *maedi-visna virus, a pathogenic lenti-retrovirus directly responsible for a chronic lymphocytic interstitial pneumonitis of sheep. In sheep with maedi, failure to thrive is often the first sign noted, followed by cough, and finally dyspnea* [difficulty breathing]. Infected sheep have enlarged lymph nodes and persistent lymphocytosis for many years. *The main histologic features of maedi infection of the lung,* a dense lymphocytic and plasma cell infiltration with areas of fibrosis, *are similar to those seen in our patients.* . . .

Further studies are needed to evaluate the role of HTLV-III/LAV in lymphocytic interstitial pneumonitis associated with AIDS and AIDS-related complex . . . [emphasis added].[25]

Interestingly, this and other studies regarding the similarities between AIDS lentivirus in humans and maedi lentivirus in sheep carefully omit mention of how the disease is spread and contained among sheep.

It is becoming increasingly obvious that the medical and media establishments are releasing piecemeal crucial facts regarding AIDS to the public. First, the public was informed that AIDS was only a disease afflicting homosexuals; now it has become an epidemic threatening to engulf the general population.

Then came the optimistic prognosis that only 5%-10% of those initially infected would come down with fatal disease. Now most experts are agreed that only a small minority, *if any*, of those infected will not face lethal consequences.

The public was bombarded with the false notion that people don't die of AIDS directly, but only from conditions associated with immune suppression. Now it is being affirmed that up to 50% or more of those infected will develop AIDS-virus induced brain disease.

In the face of this abysmal lack of understanding (or worse yet, lack of honesty) regarding this complex and fatal disease, further ongoing studies are needed to determine all potential and actual routes of AIDS spread.

FOOTNOTES

1. *Summit Journal*, March 1987.

2. L. K. Altman, "Global Program Aims to Combat AIDS Disaster", *New York Times*, 21 November 1986.

3. *Vanity Fair*, March 1987, p. 153.

4. M. A. Fischl et al., "Evaluation of Heterosexual Partners, Children, and Household Contacts of Adults with AIDS", *JAMA*, 1987; 257:640-645.

5. L. K. Altman "AIDS May Spread Outside the Blood", *New York Times*, 14 December 1986.

6. Update: "Acquired Immunodeficiency Syndrome—United States", *Morbidity and Mortality Weekly Report*, 12 December 1986.

7. Conference Report Second International Conference on the Acquired Immune Deficiency Syndrome, *Medical Journal of Australia*, 17 November 1986, p. 529.

8. K. Leishman, "Heterosexuals and AIDS", *The Atlantic Monthly*, February 1987, p. 49.

9. *MMWR*, 29 August 1986, p. 541.

10. A. C. Srivastava et al., "Identity Cards for Patients with AIDS?" *British Medical Journal*, 294; 1987:495-496.

11. P. M. Boffey, "Rights Laws Urged in AIDS Testing", *New York Times*, 25 February 1987, p. 11.

12. *MMWR*, 1986; 35:334-339.

13. Transcript from NOVA, no. 1314, "Can AIDS Be Stopped?" p. 5. WGBH Educational Foundation, Boston, Massachusetts, 1986.

14. G. Hancock and E. Carim, *AIDS The Deadly Epidemic* (London: Victor Gollancz Ltd., 1986) p. 28.

15. P.H. Black HTLV-III, "AIDS and the brain". *New England Journal of Medicine*, 1985; 313:1539-1539. A.M. Piette et al., "Acute neuropathy coincident with seroconversion for anti-HTLV-III/LAV", *Lancet*, 1986; i:852. S. Przedborski et al., "HTLV-III and vacuolar myelopathy", *New England Journal of Medicine*, 1986; 315:63.

16. D.W. Jenning et al., "Acute myelopathy associated with primary infection with human immunodeficiency virus", *British Medical Journal*, 1987; 294:143-144.

17. Jeffrey L. Madoff, Esq., "AIDS Related Employment Discrimination Issues", *AIDS Legal Aspects of a Medical Crisis* (New York: Law Journal Seminars-Press, 1986) pp. 144-145. This tome of 760 pages is an excellent resource for attorneys, legislators, actuaries, hospital boards and others dealing with legal issues involving AIDS.

18. Ibid., p. 143.

19. *New York Times*, 18 March 1986.

20. C. Neisson-Vernant et al., "Needlestick HIV Seroconversion in a Nurse". *Lancet*, 4 October 1986, p. 814.

21. R. L. Stricof and D. L. Morse, "HTLV-III/LAV Seroconversion Following a Deep Intramuscular Needlestick Injury", *New England Journal of Medicine*, 1986; 314:1115.

22. V. Wahn et al., "Horizontal transmission of HIV Infection between two siblings", *Lancet*, 20 September 1986.

23. C. J. Issel et al., "Virology of Equine Retroviruses", Chapter in *Animal Models of Retrovirus Infection and Their Relationship to AIDS*, edited by Lois Ann Salzman, Office of the Scientific Director, National Institute of Allergy and Infectious Diseases, National Institutes of Health, Bethesda, Maryland (New York: Academic Press; 1986), p. 98. See also Travis C. McGuire, "Pathogenesis of Equine Infectious Anemia", pp. 295-300 in the same work.

24. S. F. Lyons et al., "Survival of HIV in the Common Bedbug", *Lancet*, 5 July 1986, p. 45.

25. L. Resnick et al., "Detection of HTLV-III/LAV-Specific IgG and Antigen in Bronchoalveolar Lavage Fluid from Two Patients with Lymphocytic Interstitial Pneumonitis Associated with AIDS-Related Complex", *American Journal of Medicine*, 1987; 82:553-556. An addendum to the paper cites a report describing *a relatively high level of HTLV-III/LAV RNA expression by in situ hybridization* from the lung tissue of a patient with lymphocytic interstitial pneumonitis associated with AIDS. K. J. Chayt et al., "Detection of HTLV-III RNA in lungs of patients with AIDS and pulmonary involvement", *JAMA*, 1986; 256:2356-2359.

Concerned?

Concerned about the dangers posed by AIDS to you and your family? The Foundation for the Advancement of Compassion and Truth (FACT) is a valuable resource. FACT publishes a monthly newsletter keeping readers updated with current information. The newsletter also includes timely suggestions for personal, community and legislative action.

FACT appreciates letters, articles (please include source and date) and questions. If a personal response is desired, please enclose a self-addressed envelope. (Information from medical and legal professionals is especially welcomed.)

FACT newsletter subscription: $25.00 per year

Audio cassette by Gene Antonio, along with the report "A Critical Evaluation of the Surgeon-General's Report on AIDS": $6.95 (includes postage)

Make check or money order payable to:

> FACT
> 4101 Green Oaks Blvd. West
> Suite 264
> Arlington, TX 76016